DIAGNOSTIC PICTURE TESTS IN

Clinical Infectious Diseases

Nick

MA, FRCP, ~~~~~ DTM&H
Senior Lecturer ...ectious Diseases
Liverpool School of Tropical Medicine
Liverpool, UK

Fred J. Nye
MD, FRCP
Clinical Director
Infectious Disease Unit
Fazakerley Hospital
Liverpool, UK

⋀ Mosby-Wolfe

London Baltimore Barcelona Bogotá Boston Buenos Aires Caracas Carlsbad, CA Chicago Madrid Mexico City
Milan Naples, FL New York Philadelphia St. Louis Seoul Singapore Sydney Taipei Tokyo Toronto Wiesbaden

Titles published in the Diagnostic Picture Tests series include:

Picture Tests in Human Anatomy
DPT in Cardiology
DPT in Clinical Medicine,
DPT in Clinical Neurology
DPT in Clinical Surgery
DPT in Dentistry
DPT in Dermatology
DPT in Ear, Nose and Throat
DPT in Embryology, 2nd edn
DPT in Endocrinology, 2nd edn
DPT in Gastroenterology
DPT in General Medicine, Vols 1–4
DPT in General Surgery
DPT in Geriatric Medicine
DPT in Infectious Disease

DPT in Injury and Sport
DPT in Obstetrics and Gynecology
DPT in Ophthalmology
DPT in Oral Medicine
DPT in Orthopedics
DPT in Pediatrics, 2nd edn
DPT in Pediatric Dermatology
DPT in Pediatric Dentistry
DPT in Respiratory Disease
DPT in Rheumatology
Differential Diagnosis in AIDS
DPT in Urology
400 Self Assessment PictureTests in
    Clinical Medicine
400 More Self Assessment Picture Tests
    in Clinical Medicine

Project Manager:	Alison Taylor
Cover Design:	Lara Last
Layout Artist:	Lindy van den Berghe
Production:	Jane Tozer
Index:	Jill Halliday
Publisher:	Jennifer Prast

Copyright © 1996 Times Mirror International Publishers Limited

Published in 1996 by Mosby-Wolfe, an imprint of Times Mirror International Publishers Limited

Printed in Italy by Vincenzo Bona s.r.l., Turin

ISBN 0 7234 2451 9

Warning
The doses of pharmaceutical products given in this book are a guide only. Although every effort is made to ensure accuracy, the authors and publishers cannot be held responsible for the accuracy of these dosages. It is recommended that the reader, if in doubt, checks the latest editions of publications such as the British National Formulary, Martindale's Extra Pharmacopoeia or MIMS (Monthly Index of Medical Specialities).

Preface

The management of clinical infection cuts across the boundaries of system-related specialities, and is as important in the community as in hospital practice. This collection of photographs has been compiled to illustrate the range of infections that may be encountered in the developed world, and includes common presentations of some imported infections. Most of the cases are relatively straightforward and we anticipate that the book will be of use to medical students, postgraduates studying for examinations such as the MRCP and MRCPath, and for general practitioners.

Nick Beeching
Fred Nye

Acknowledgements

We are pleased to thank our publishers for their enthusiasm and guidance, especially Jennifer Prast and Alison Taylor. We also thank Jean Taylor and Val Robbins for typing and organising the manuscript. Many of the photographs were taken by Richard Hancock of the Department of Medical Illustration, Aintree Hospitals NHS Trust and by Graham Watson, Department of Medical Illustration, Liverpool School of Tropical Medicine. We also acknowledge the Departments of Medical Illustration at East Birmingham Hospital (now Birmingham Heartlands Hospital), Auckland Hospital and Middlemore Hospital (Auckland, New Zealand) and the Royal Liverpool University Hospital.

We are grateful to many of our colleagues for providing or allowing us to use illustrations of patients admitted under their care: Dr LK Archibald, Dr Ashfak Ahmad, Dr OP Arya, Dr JW Bailey, Dr DR Bell, Dr JS Cheesbrough, Dr AB Christie, Mrs J Duvall-Young, Dr RB Ellis-Pegler, Professor AM Geddes, Dr CF Gilks, Dr GV Gill, Professor AD Harries, Professor CA Hart, Dr Rizwan Ullah Khan, Dr JA Innes, Dr RD Isaacs, Dr SDR Lang, Dr D Maher, Dr JH Martindale, Professor HV Morgan, Dr CJ Parry, Dr E Rodrigues, Dr PJ Southall, Dr W Taylor, Dr C Valentine, Dr GB Wyatt.

We specifically acknowledge the following for permission to reproduce illustrations that have been previously published elsewhere:
Centre for Applied Microbiology and Research, Porton Down, Salisbury, Wiltshire, UK – figure 88.
Infectious Diseases: Epidemiology and Clinical Practice, AB Christie, 4th Edition 1987. Churchill Livingstone, Edinburgh, UK – figures 19, 30, 96, 132.
The Director, *Center for Disease Control and Prevention (CDC),* National Center for Infectious Diseases, Fort Collins, Colorado, USA – figure 74.
International Diabetes Digest, FSG Communications Ltd, Reach, Cambridgeshire, UK – figure 121.
Liverpool School of Tropical Medicine, Liverpool, UK – figure 83.
World Health Organization, Geneva, Switzerland – figures 29, 132.

Finally, we apologise if any colleagues or publishers have inadvertantly been omitted.

1 ▶

This 65-year-old man from the Middle East presented with two months of weight loss and abdominal discomfort. The bag contains ascitic fluid.

a) What are the possible diagnoses?
b) How would you investigate him?
c) What is his prognosis?

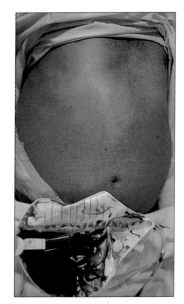

2 ▶

This woman suffered from severe cellulitis of the left leg. A few months earlier she had had a left hip replacement.

a) What organisms may be responsible for the cellulitis?
b) How may a bacteriological diagnosis be made?
c) Why is this patient at special risk?

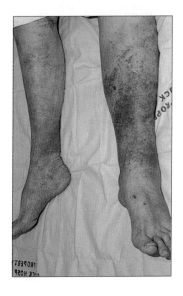

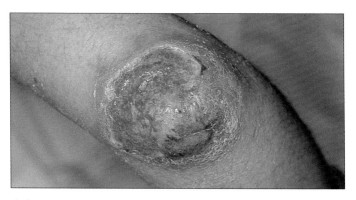

▲ 3

This young man had been backpacking in Bolivia and Brazil and presented with this ulcer, which had developed on his elbow over a period of 2 months.

a) What are the possible diagnoses?

b) How would you investigate?

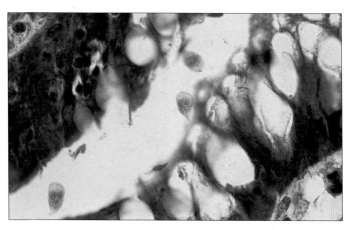

▲ 4

This is a high power view (modified trichrome) of a jejunal biopsy from a young man with chronic diarrhea and negative fecal microscopy.

a) What is the diagnosis?

b) How else could it have been diagnosed?

5 ▶

This 25-year-old drug abuser had been treated for a right pleural effusion 2 years previously. He presented with progressive low back pain and sciatica.

a) What is the most likely diagnosis of the lesions shown on the a-p spine view (upper) and the MR scan (lower)?

b) How should it be investigated?

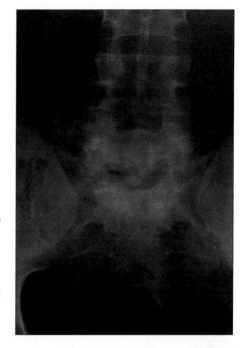

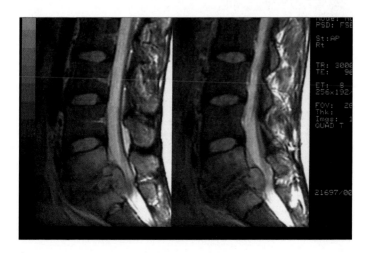

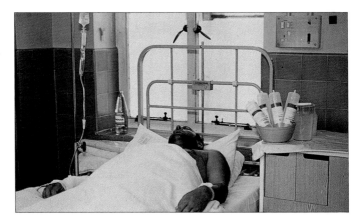

▲ 6

This man developed profuse watery diarrhea while flying from the Indian subcontinent to Britain, and was admitted to hospital on arrival. His IV and oral fluid requirements for 2 hours are shown.
a) What is the diagnosis?
b) How would you confirm it?

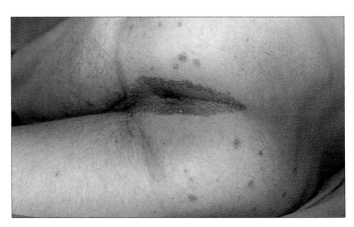

▲ 7

This married engineer had worked in several countries in Africa for 10 years and presented with fever and weight loss for 2 months.
a) What skin lesion is demonstrated?
b) What other diagnoses might you think of?

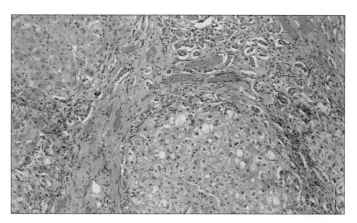

▲ 8

This medium power photo micrograph (hematoxylin and eosin) is of the liver of a patient who was an HIV positive hemophiliac.
a) What abnormalities are present?
b) What is the likely etiology?

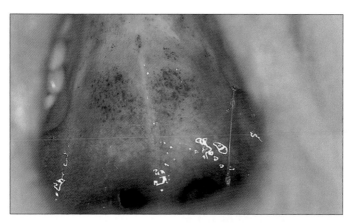

▲ 9

The patient complained of fever, malaise and myalgia. On examination he had generalized lymphadenopathy.
a) What is shown in the photograph?
b) What virus infections may be responsible?

5

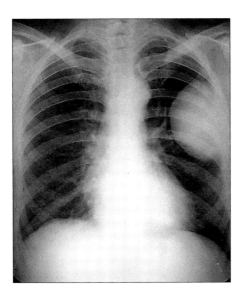

◀ **10**

This asymptomatic patient was brought up in a rural part of Wales and the radiographic findings were incidental.

a) What are the possible diagnoses?

b) What is the usual primary host of the etiological agent?

c) What is the natural history?

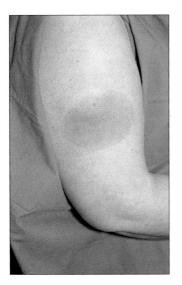

◀ **11**

The patient complained that the site of a recent tetanus toxoid booster immunization had become painful.

What action is required?

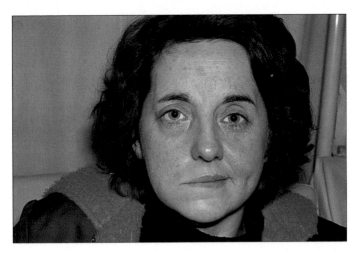

▲ 12
What infections are associated with this neurological abnormality?

13 ▶
This man from the Middle East has a hole in his hard palate in addition to the abnormality shown.
a) What is the differential diagnosis?
b) What serological tests might be useful?

Syphillis

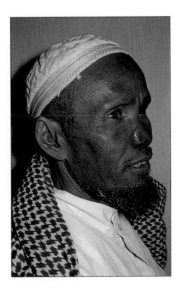

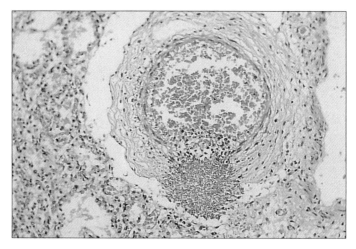

▲ 14

This medium power micrograph (hematoxylin and eosin) shows a blood vessel in the lung of a baby who died after 3 weeks of total parenteral nutrition in intensive care.

a) What does it show?
b) What other stains might be useful?

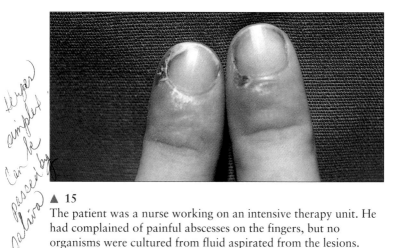

▲ 15

The patient was a nurse working on an intensive therapy unit. He had complained of painful abscesses on the fingers, but no organisms were cultured from fluid aspirated from the lesions. What is the likely causative organism and how should it be treated?

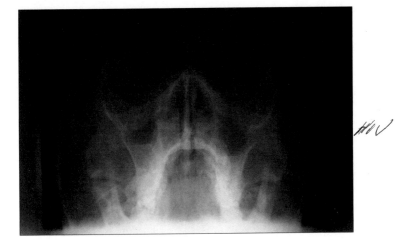

HIV

▲ 16

This HIV positive woman presented with short lived facial pain and fever.

a) What abnormalities are present?

b) What are the most likely pathogens?

17 ▶

This 30-foot-long specimen was passed per rectum by a physician after treatment for "worms" acquired after a conference in Finland.

a) What is the "worm"?

b) How is it acquired?

c) What problems can occur in infected individuals?

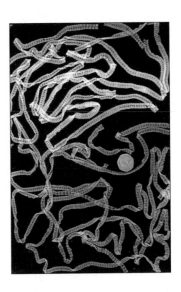

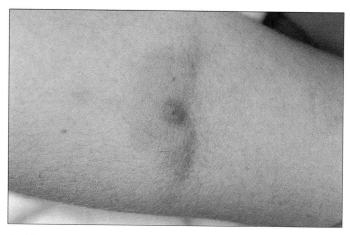

▲ 18

A 35-year-old woman presented with low grade fever and recurrent mouth ulcers. Six months before she had been admitted to hospital with lymphocytic meningitis from which she had recovered.
a) What phenomenon is illustrated in her antecubital fossa?
b) What is the likely diagnosis?

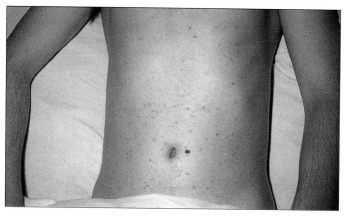

▲ 19

This young man returned from a holiday in Indonesia complaining of fever and abdominal pain.
What is the diagnosis?

(See acknowledgements)

20 ▶
The patient had chickenpox. What are the risk factors for the complication shown?

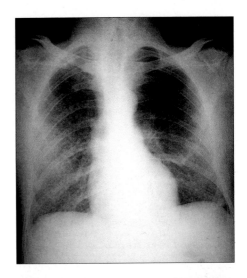

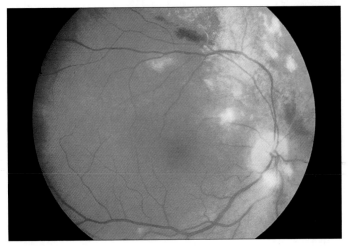

▲ 21
The patient was HIV positive and had a CD4 count of 50 cells/ml
a) What is the likely diagnosis?
b) How is this diagnosis established?
c) What other organs or tissues may be affected in HIV infected individuals?

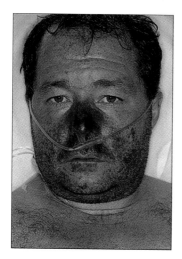

◀ 22
This patient was admitted to hospital as an emergency with suspected septicemia. Ten years previously he had had a laparotomy because of abdominal trauma.
a) What is the likely diagnosis?
b) How might it have been prevented?

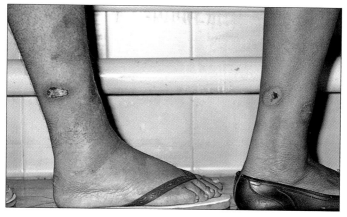

▲ 23
These two men from North India were hospitalized in the same ward for treatment of the same condition.
a) What abnormalities are present?
b) What were their diagnoses?
c) What other physical signs might be present?

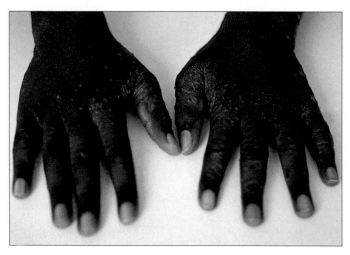

▲ 24

This patient had lymphadenopathy, splenomegaly and itching of the hands.
a) What is the probable diagnosis?
b) What is the underlying diagnosis?

25 ▶

The painful lesions shown had developed over a period of 2 weeks.
a) What etiologies would you consider?
b) How would you treat the patient?

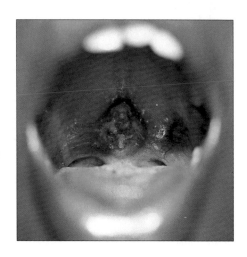

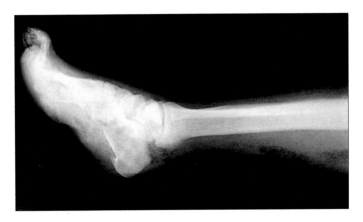

▲ 26
a) What abnormality is present in this X-ray?
b) What underlying condition might be present?

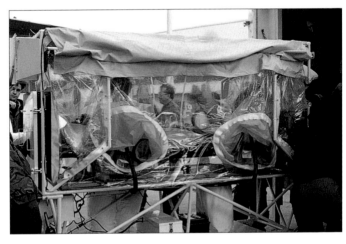

▲ 27
What infections might justify the use of this equipment?

28 ▶

a) What is the diagnosis?
b) How may it be rapidly
   confirmed?

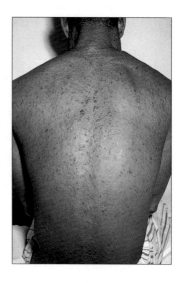

29 ▶

This young Indonesian man has
had weakness and deformity of
the right arm and hand since
the age of four.
a) What is the diagnosis?
b) Is the deformity preventable?
(See Acknowledgements)

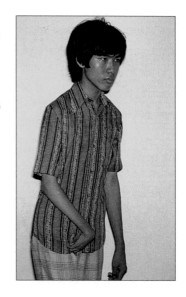

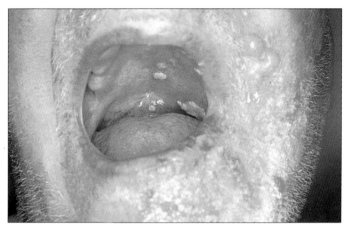

▲ 30
This patient had a painful skin eruption on the face.
What is the diagnosis and what complication has occurred?
(See acknowledgements)

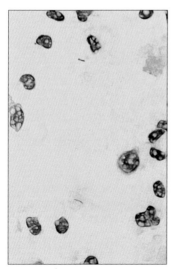

◄ 31
The patient was an 81-year-old woman who had suffered from recurrent urinary tract infections and persistent pyuria. Her GP asked for a diagnostic procedure to be carried out on a specimen of urine.

a) What is shown in the stained smear of centrifuged urinary deposit?

b) How may the condition predispose to recurrent urinary tract infection?

32 ▶

This 35-year-old IV drug user
had impairment of short-term
memory.
a) What does the scan show?
b) What is the likely cause?
c) How might it be treated?

HIV –
Caused dementia –
mental confusion

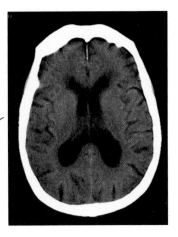

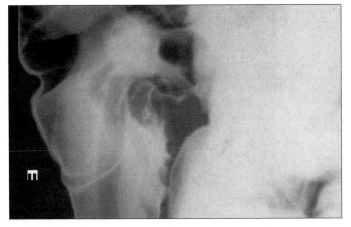

▲ **33**

A 38-year-old man with AIDS presented with 3 weeks of tenderness
in the right iliac fossa, mild diarrhea and "floaters" in his vision.
a) What abnormality is present in the caecum?
b) What is the most likely cause?
c) What non-invasive part of the physical examination is essential?

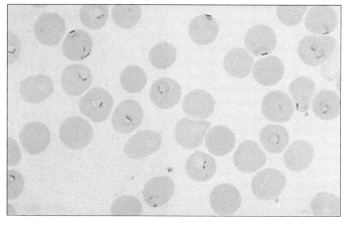

▲ 34

This patient presented with fever two weeks after returning from a holiday in Zimbabwe. She had taken malaria prophylaxis.
a) What is the diagnosis?
b) What are the key hematological features distinguishing this from similar infections?

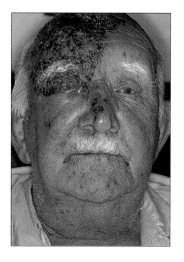

◄ 35
a) What complications may affect this patient's eye?
b) Why is he particularly at risk from eye involvement?

36 ▶

Both these men presented with fever, headache and mild diarrhea 4 weeks after returning from Bangkok.

a) What diagnoses would you consider?

b) What serological tests are indicated?

HIV

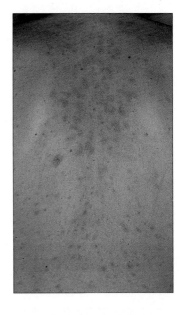

Syphilis

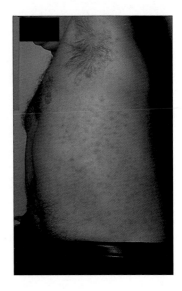

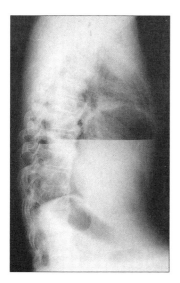

◀ 37
a) What is shown on this lateral chest X-ray?
b) What organisms are likely to be recovered from this lesion?

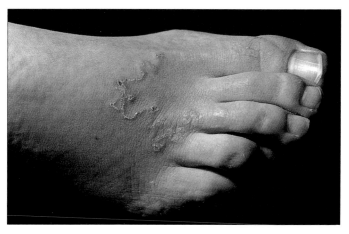

▲ 38
The itchy lesion shown had been present for two weeks, shortly after a visit to a Caribbean resort.
a) What is the diagnosis?
b) How is it treated?

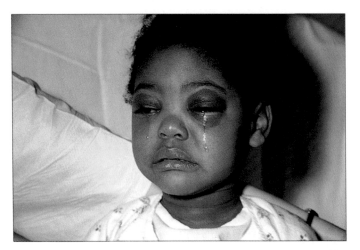

▲ 39

This child had a severe paroxysmal cough.
a) What is the likely cause of the cough?
b) What is the abnormality shown and how is it caused?

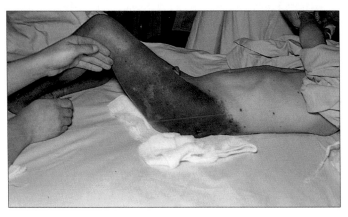

▲ 40

The patient had mild chickenpox with a sparse rash.
What life threatening complication has developed, and what is the pathogenesis?

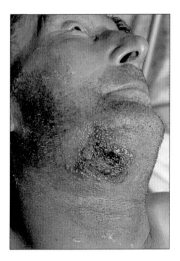

◀ 41

This man had been handling imported hides.

a) What is the likely cause of the skin lesion?

b) What rapid test can be done to confirm the diagnosis?

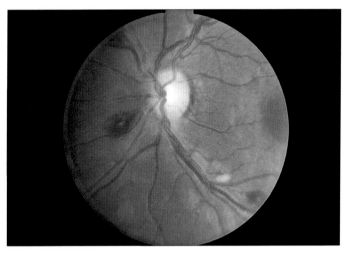

▲ 42

A young woman developed rigors for 4 days and on admission had fever and anemia.

a) What abnormalities are present in her optic fundus?

b) What is the unifying diagnosis?

c) What are the most likely organisms involved?

43 ▶

This Pakistani man had a 7-day history of nausea, tiredness, pale feces and vague fever.

a) What is the likely etiology of his jaundice?
b) What are the most important initial investigations?

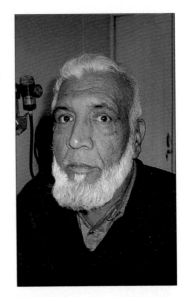

44 ▶

A 32-year-old man had a sudden focal seizure while returning from a holiday in Florida. He then developed fever, a fluctuating level of consciousness, dysphasia and a right hemiplegia.

a) What is the diagnosis?
b) How is the diagnosis established?
c) How should the patient be treated?

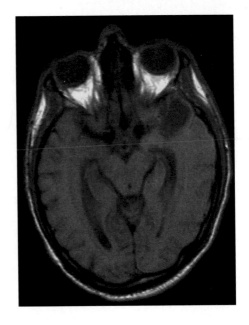

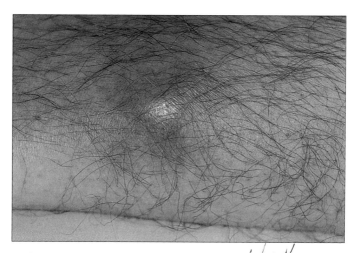

▲ 45

The patient had advanced HIV infection.

HIV

What is the differential diagnosis of this painful lesion on the leg?

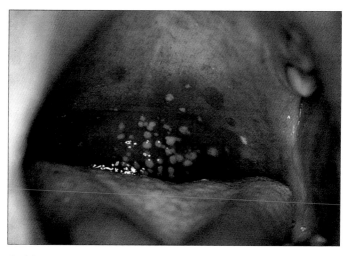

▲ 46

What is this condition and what organisms are responsible?

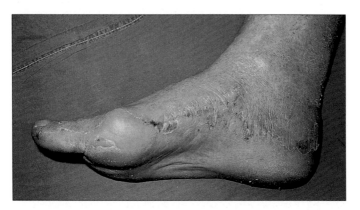

▲ 47

a) What is this common skin complaint?

b) How is it diagnosed and treated?

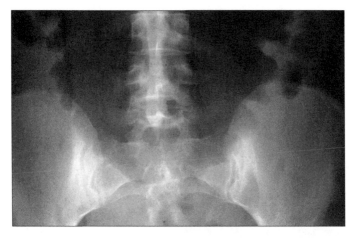

▲ 48

The patient had a history of 1 week of bloody diarrhea. She had been treated with oral amoxycillin.

a) What is shown on the abdominal X-ray?

b) What is the differential diagnosis?

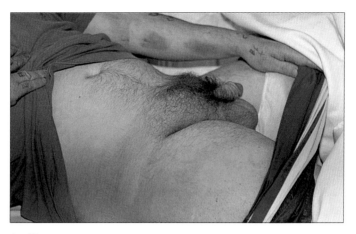

▲ 49
The patient illustrated had recently injected heroin into his groin.
a) What complications have arisen?
b) What investigations are needed?

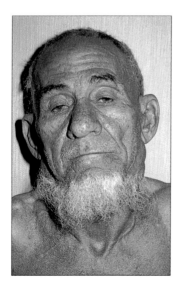

◄ 50
This man with long-standing chronic lymphatic leukemia came back early to the clinic with fever and painful enlargement of his neck glands. What investigations are indicated?

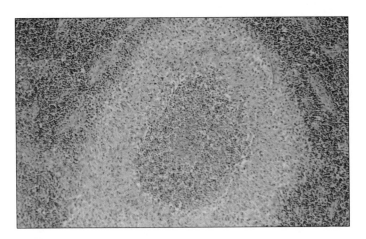

▲ 51

The high power view illustrates a lesion in the appendix (hematoxylin and eosin) removed from a young farmer with abdominal pain.

a) What is illustrated?
b) What treatment is indicated?

52 ▶

A 25-year-old woman developed tingling in her feet and rapidly became unable to walk. The chart shows her respiratory rate (RR) and vital capacity (VC) from day 5 of her illness.

a) What is the diagnosis?
b) What infectious causes have been implicated?
c) What treatment is indicated?

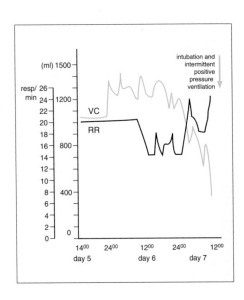

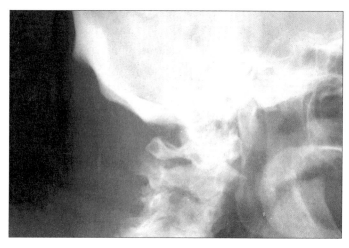

▲ 53

The X-rays illustrated were taken after a British man presented with a focal seizure. He had lived in India for 2 years, returning to Britain 7 years previously.

a) What do the X-rays show?
b) What is the infecting organism?
c) How would you treat him?

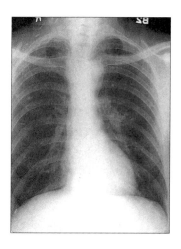

54 ▶

The painful lesions illustrated developed over 10 days, spreading from small "spots" Four months later the patient developed bloody diarrhea.

a) What is the diagnosis?

b) What is the connection with the bloody diarrhea?

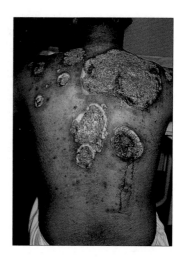

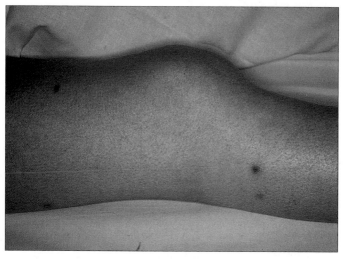

▲ **55**

The painless papular lesions demonstrated were associated with fever, 10 days after a bone marrow transplantation.

a) What is the diagnosis?

b) What is the treatment?

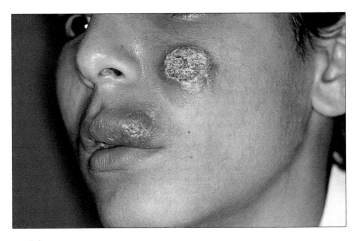

▲ 56
This Pakistani boy had developed the lesion shown over 3 weeks.
a) What is the diagnosis?
b) What treatment is indicated?

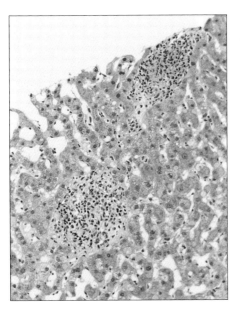

◀ 57
A 30-year-old man from the Middle East had intermittent fever, mild anemia and thrombocytopenia and slightly raised transaminase levels.
a) What does the liver biopsy show?
b) What other investigations might help?

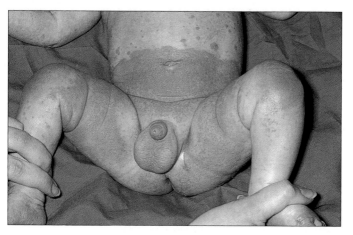

▲ 58
a) What is the cause of this common rash?
b) How should it be treated?

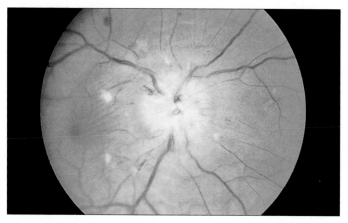

▲ 59
The patient, who was HIV positive, presented with fever, headache, confusion and these fundal appearances.
a) What is the likely diagnosis?
b) What confirmatory investigations are necessary?

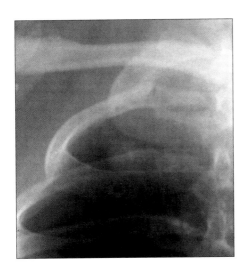

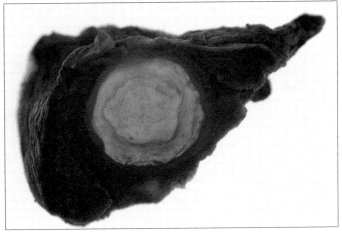

▲ 60

This woman in her fifties had an asymptomatic lesion shown in the apical chest tomogram (upper); the 2 cm lesion was resected (lower) to exclude malignancy. No other lesions were seen on the chest X-ray.

a) What infectious diagnoses would you consider?

b) What pointers might be obtained from the history?

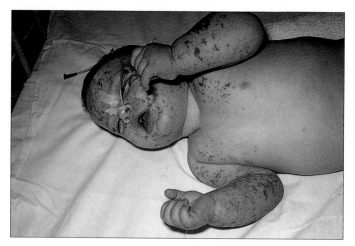

▲ 61

This infant was referred to a casualty department with the provisional diagnosis of child abuse.

a) What signs are present?

b) What is the most likely diagnosis?

c) What immediate treatment is required?

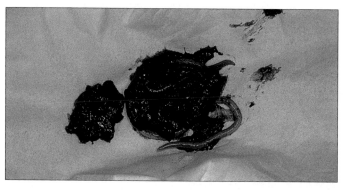

▲ 62

The above fecal specimen was produced by a child who had recently arrived in Britain from the Indian subcontinent.

a) What pathogen is present?

b) How should it be treated?

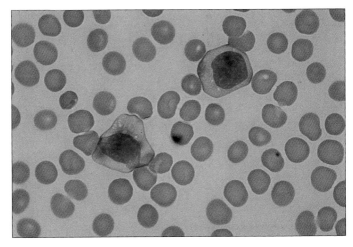

▲ 63
a) In what common infection are these cells seen in the peripheral blood?
b) What are these cells, and what is their function?

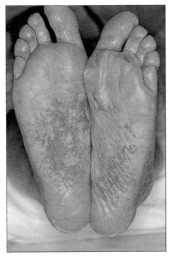

◄ 64
This patient had severe vasculitis affecting the skin and the cerebral and renal vasculature.
What infection may underlie this condition?

a) What is this condition?
b) Under what circumstances does it affect young children?

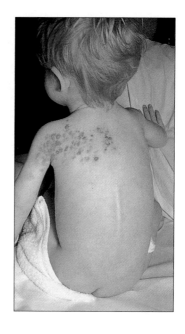

The patient complained of a severe sore throat and was febrile with enlarged posterior cervical lymph nodes. She had not received any antibiotic therapy.
What is the diagnosis?

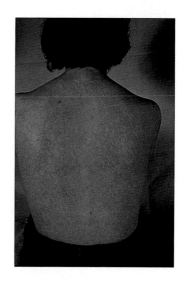

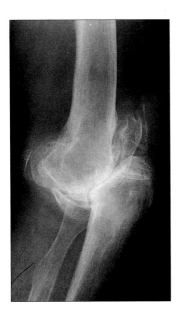

◄ 67

An 87-year-old woman had a deformed knee (upper) and X-rays of her pelvic area (lower) yielded further clues to her past medical history.

a) What abnormalities are present in the radiograph?
b) What is the unifying diagnosis?

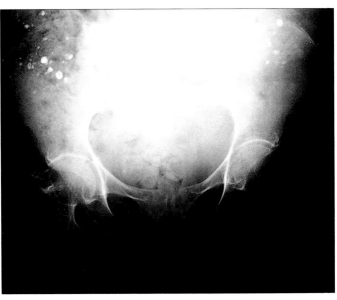

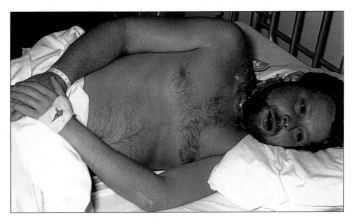

▲ 68

This wind-surfer presented to the emergency room with headache and fever.

a) What other abnormalities are present?

b) What is the diagnosis?

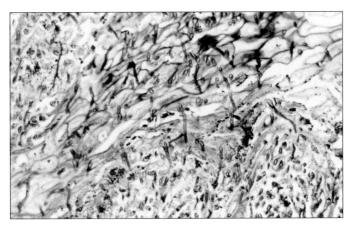

▲ 69

This is a medium power view (Grocott stain) of a biopsy of the lower esophagus from a patient with discomfort on swallowing.

a) What does it show?

b) What are possible predisposing factors?

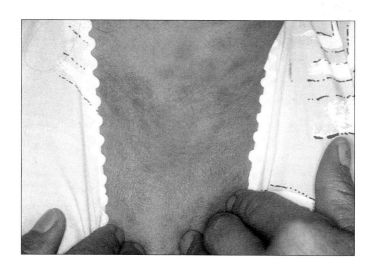

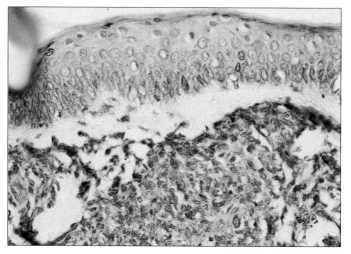

▲ 70

A middle aged woman from India presented with a chronic rash on her chest (upper). A low power view of a skin biopsy from her arm is shown (lower).

a) What is the diagnosis?

b) Is she infectious to others?

71 ▶

The patient had emergency surgery for debridement of extensive subcutaneous gangrene, which had started initially as a small septic lesion on the scrotum.

a) What is the diagnosis?
b) What organisms are responsible?
c) How should the infection be managed?

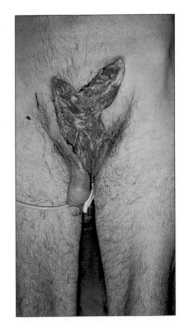

72 ▶

This woman had an abdominal aortic aneurysm successfully treated with an aortic prosthetic graft. Ten years later she presented with intermittent fever and pain and redness of both ankles.

What is shown in the CT scan of her abdomen?

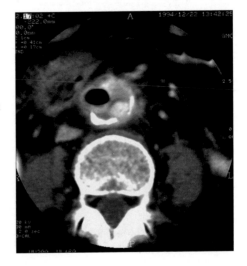

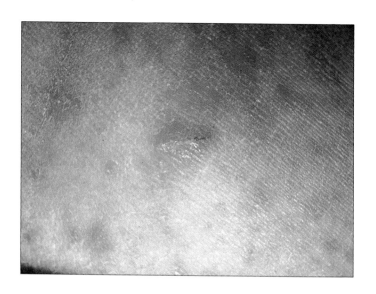

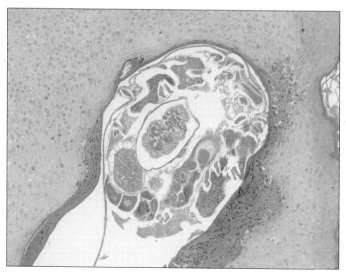

▲ 73
This pruritic rash (upper) was biopsied (lower).
What is the diagnosis and what treatment is indicated?

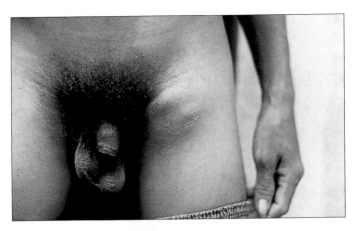

▲ 74

This patient presented during an epidemic, with sudden onset of fever and enlarged tender inguinal glands.

What infection should be suspected and how may the diagnosis be confirmed?

(See acknowledgements)

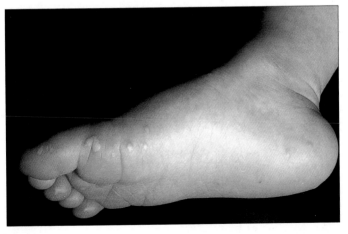

▲ 75

As well as these lesions on the extremities, the patient had a vesicular stomatitis.

What is the diagnosis and what is the cause?

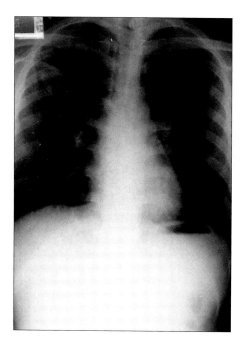

◀ 76
The patient was a
Hong Kong
resident. He
presented with
fever, headache and
mental confusion.
What is the likely
diagnosis?

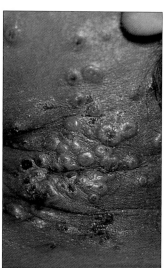

◀ 77
The patient had secondary
infection of eczematous skin.
What is the differential
diagnosis?

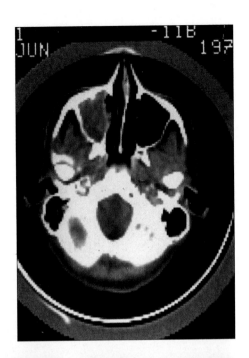

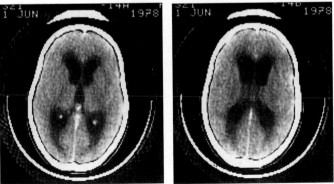

▲ 78

The patient was a young woman with severe pneumococcal meningitis.

a) What is the source of the meningeal infection (upper)?

b) What complication ensued (lower)?

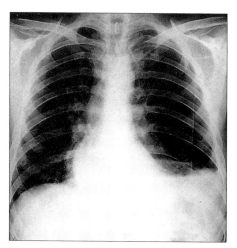

◄ 79
A young man presented to the emergency room with fever for 3 days followed by abrupt onset of chest pain and dyspnea.
a) What abnormalities are present in this chest X-ray?
b) What causes would you consider?

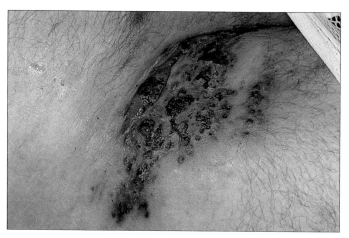

▲ 80
This vascular skin tumor had been treated with superficial radiotherapy. The lesions were ulcerated and there was much bruising, edema and secondary infection.
a) What is the diagnosis?
b) How should the lesion be treated initially?

81 ▶

The patient had had extensive surgery for colonic carcinoma involving the bladder. What complication has occurred?

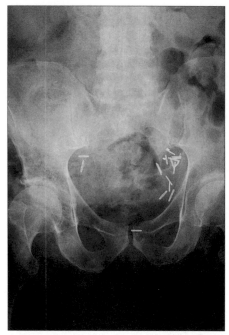

82 ▶

The patient was an 18-year-old woman who had noticed mild disturbance of vision one year previously.

a) What is the probable diagnosis?
b) Would serological tests be useful?
c) What treatment is required?

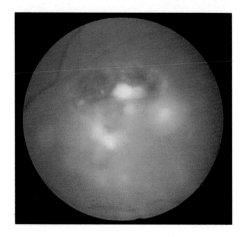

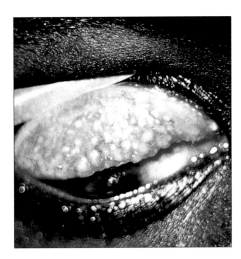

◄ 83

This man from West Africa complained of a gritty sensation in his eyes for several years.
a) What is the diagnosis?
b) What is the causative organism?
c) What is the treatment?

(See Acknowledgements)

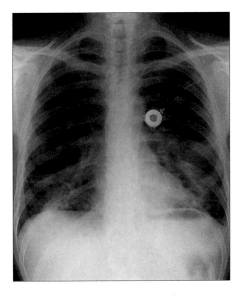

◄ 84

This man with AIDS had been on treatment for CMV retinitis for 7 months. Over the past month he had increased malaise and a chronic non-productive cough.
a) What is the likely cause?
b) What investigations would help?

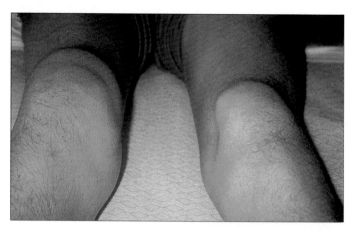

▲ 85
The patient developed painful joints after a diarrheal illness.
a) What bacterial pathogens are associated with it?
b) What is the predisposing genetic factor?

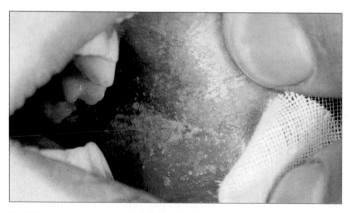

▲ 86
This child was febrile and miserable with marked coryzal symptoms. Four days later a skin rash started on the face and spread rapidly to the rest of the body.
What is the diagnosis, and what are the mouth lesions?

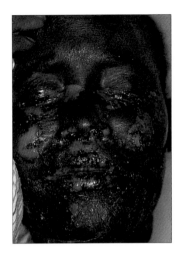

◀ 87
This African woman recently started treatment for tuberculosis.
a) What are the diagnoses?
b) What are the most likely causes?

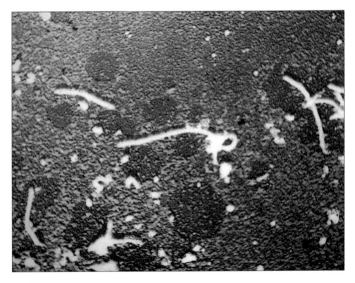

▲ 88
a) What type of virus is shown in the electron micrograph?
b) What human diseases are caused by this group of agents?

(See Acknowledgements)

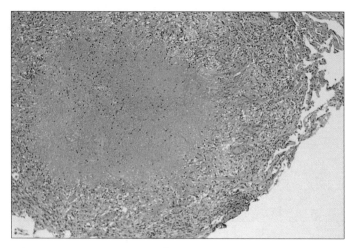

▲ 89

A 45-year-old man underwent a transbronchial biopsy because of cough and fever.

a) What does the biopsy show? (low power, hematoxylin and eosin)

b) What is the diagnosis?

90 ▶

This radiograph was taken prior to intravenous urography. The patient had had recurrent urinary tract infection for many years.

a) What abnormalities are present?

b) What is the most likely urinary pathogen?

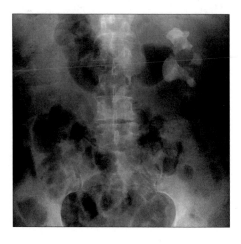

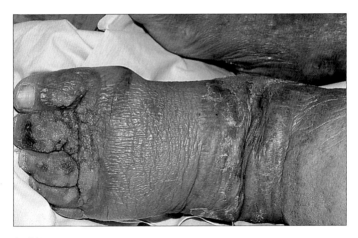

▲ 91
This middle aged Samoan man had chronic leg problems and was admitted in a shocked state with fever of 24 hours' duration.
a) What is the etiology of his leg problems?
b) What has caused his recent illness?

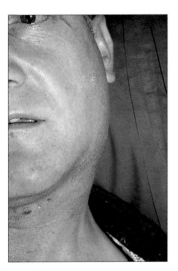

◀ 92
A few days after this photograph was taken the patient had a series of major seizures and became severely obtunded.
What is the diagnosis?

93 ▶

A week after returning from holiday in southern Spain this patient became febrile and was disorientated in time and space. His illness failed to respond to amoxycillin.

a) What is the differential diagnosis?
b) What diagnostic tests should be performed?

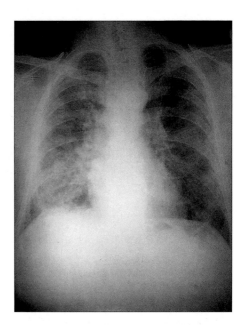

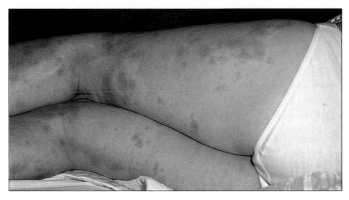

▲ 94

a) What is this skin condition?
b) One week before the skin changes appeared the patient suffered from a diarrheal illness. What was its likely cause?

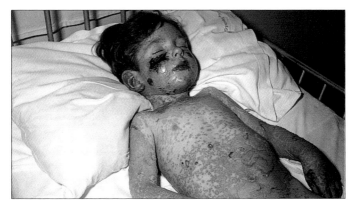

▲ 95
This child suffered from blistering skin lesions which left a raw weeping surface.
a) What common bacterial pathogen causes this syndrome?
b) What is the syndrome called?
c) What is the pathogenesis?

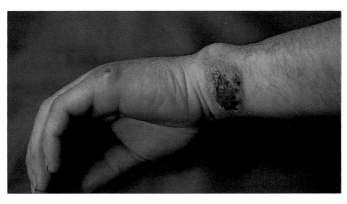

▲ 96
A sheep farmer complained of these painless vesicular lesions on the hand and wrist.
a) What is the cause of the lesions?
b) How may the condition be diagnosed?
c) What treatment is indicated?
(See acknowledgements)

97 ▶

A Pakistani sailor presented to an emergency room with right sided pleuritic chest pain. After a chest X-ray (upper) he was discharged with a prescription for amoxycillin. A few days later he returned with severe right sided pain, and the X-ray appearances shown (lower).

a) What changes are shown on X-ray?

b) What is the likely diagnosis?

c) What further investigations are necessary?

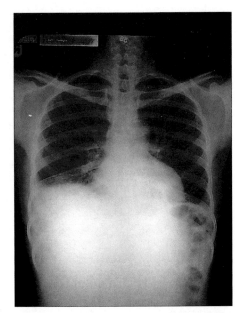

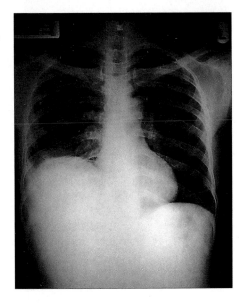

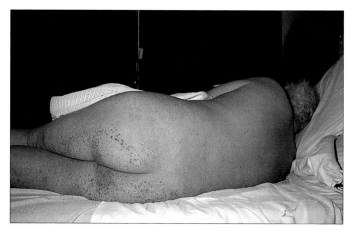

▲ 98

The skin lesions were raised, and did not fade on pressure.

a) What is the condition?

b) What infection may trigger it?

c) What are the possible complications?

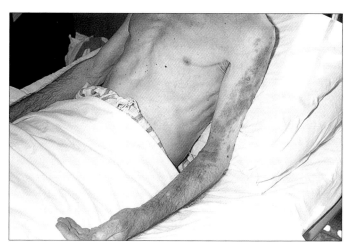

▲ 99

a) What is shown here?

b) What common complications may follow?

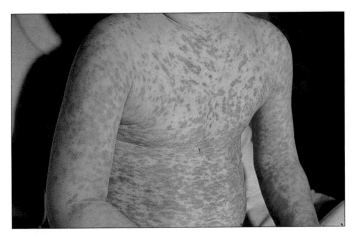

▲ 100
This child had a heavy "cold" which had been treated with amoxycillin.
What are the diagnostic possibilities?

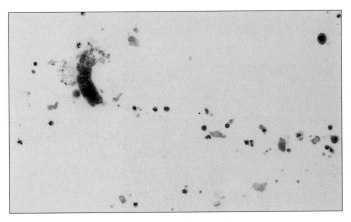

▲ 101
The patient was a consultant pathologist who complained of hematuria two weeks after recovery from a sore throat.
a) What is shown in the centrifuged urinary deposit?
b) What bacteriological investigations are necessary?

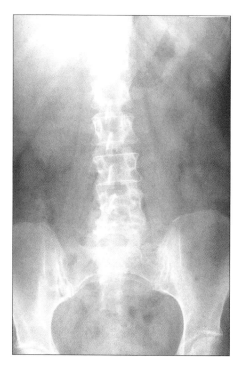

A 60-year-old woman was investigated in clinic for recurrent hypotension and vomiting.

a) What do the plain abdominal film (upper) and CT scan (lower) of her upper abdomen show?

b) What is the likely diagnosis and cause?

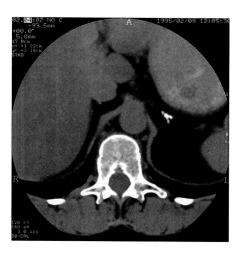

56

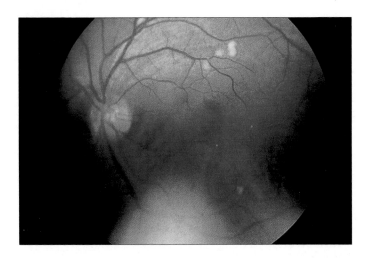

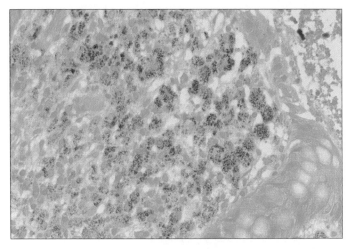

▲ 103

A 32-year-old man developed intermittent fever, sweats and diarrhea. After a month, fundoscopy showed the lesion in the upper figure, and a rectal biopsy was taken (lower). He had had 2 previous episodes of *Pneumocystis carinii* pneumonia.

a) What type of stain has been used in the lower figure?

b) What is the likely diagnosis?

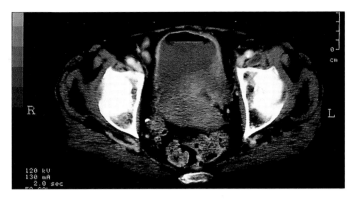

▲ 104

A 67-year-old woman developed intermittent rigors and *Enterococcus fecalis* and *Bacteroides fragilis* were isolated from blood cultures.

a) What does the CT scan of her lower pelvis show?
b) What other typical symptoms might she have?

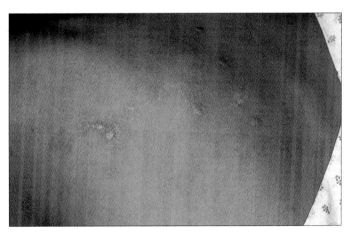

▲ 105

This young woman from Central Africa presented with smear positive pulmonary tuberculosis.

a) What abnormality is present on her shoulder?
b) What is its significance?

106 ►

This man developed high fever shortly after chemotherapy for leukemia. The lesion on his arm developed after he was given a neutrophil-rich transfusion to correct severe neutropenia.

a) What is this lesion called?

b) What organism was cultured from it?

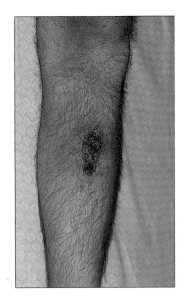

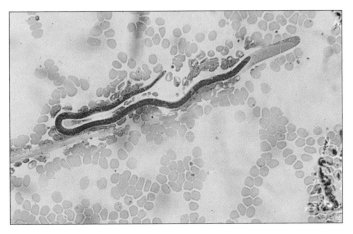

▲ 107

This Giemsa-stained blood film was taken from an asymptomatic Samoan woman with eosinophilia detected in late pregnancy.

a) What does it show?

b) How could it be treated?

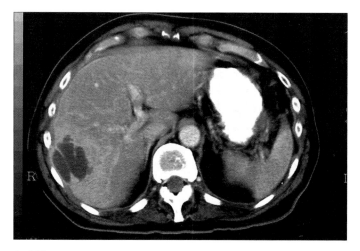

▲ 108

A 45-year old-man was admitted for investigation of fever without localizing signs.

a) What does the enhanced CT scan show?

b) What is the likely organism?

c) What is the likely origin?

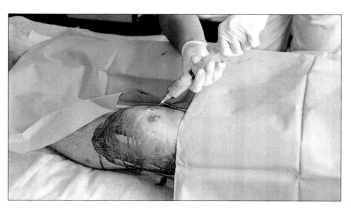

▲ 109

The diagnostic knee aspiration was performed on a drug abuser.

a) What investigations are required?

b) What further management is indicated?

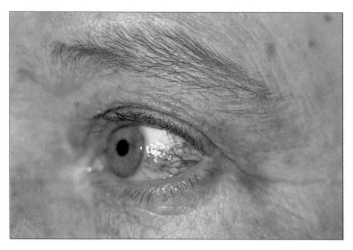

▲ 110

What systemic infection is associated with this unusual type of conjunctivitis?

111 ▶

A 57-year-old man presented with fever, jaundice and mental confusion. Mitral systolic and diastolic murmurs were audible.

a) What is the diagnosis?

b) What complication is responsible for his mental confusion?

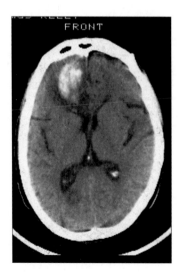

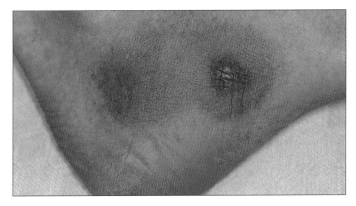

▲ 112

An intensely itchy lesion appeared on this patient's ankle while she was being treated for a urinary tract infection. She gave a history of a similar skin eruption which had appeared on the same ankle 6 months previously, under almost exactly the same circumstances. What is the likely cause of the skin lesion?

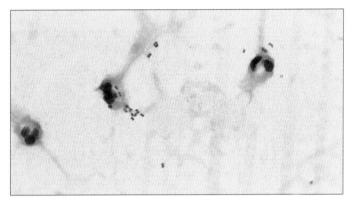

▲ 113

The photograph shows a Gram-stained smear of CSF obtained from a 16-year-old boy with acute meningitis.

a) What is the bacteriological diagnosis?

b) What infection control measures should be taken?

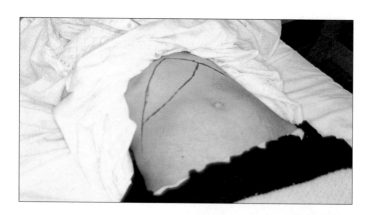

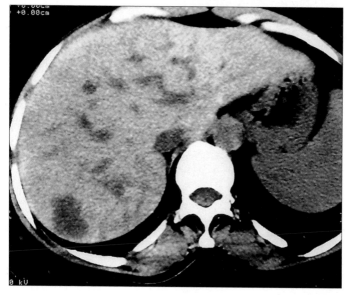

▲ 114

This woman (upper) had recently arrived in Britain from the Middle East and had an enlarged, tender liver, low grade fever and eosinophilia.

a) What abnormality is shown in the un-enhanced CT scan (lower) of her upper abdomen?

b) What is the likely diagnosis?

c) What other investigations might help?

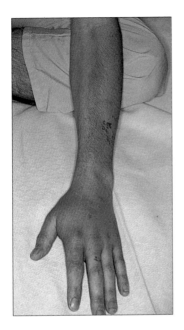

◀ 115
The patient had injected temazepam into his hand.
a) What phenomenon is illustrated?
b) What is the likely infecting organism?

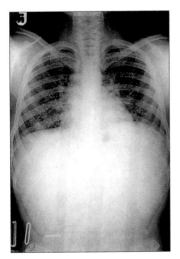

◀ 116
This boy had a febrile illness 3 years before the chest X-ray illustrated was taken.
a) What is shown?
b) What was his illness 3 years ago?

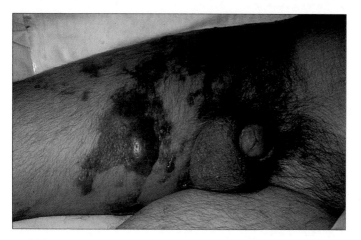

▲ 117

The patient developed exquisite local pain 12 hours before the above rash appeared, in association with hypotension.

a) What is the diagnosis?

b) How should he be treated?

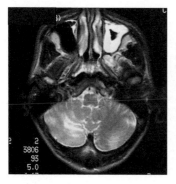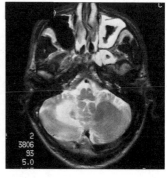

▲ 118

This MR scan was obtained when a 42-year-old man with AIDS developed forgetfulness and difficulty walking.

a) What does it show?

b) What diagnoses would you consider?

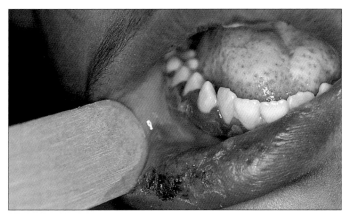

▲ 119

This young man had severe mouth pain and foul breath.

a) What is the diagnosis?

b) How should he be treated?

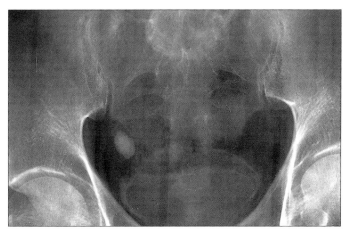

▲ 120

This plain abdominal film was taken prior to intravenous urography. The patient had lived in the Middle East.

a) What does it show?

b) What is the diagnosis and treatment?

121 ▶

This diabetic patient presented with severe facial pain.

a) What diagnoses would you consider?

b) What investigations are required?

(See acknowledgements)

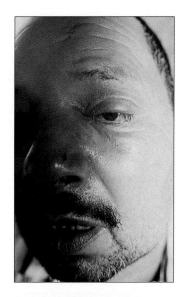

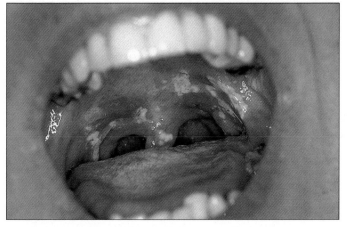

▲ **122**

This 32-year-old man complained of malaise, severe fatigue and weight loss. Chest X-ray revealed bilateral nodular shadows.

a) What is causing the appearances in the pharynx?

b) What is the underlying diagnosis?

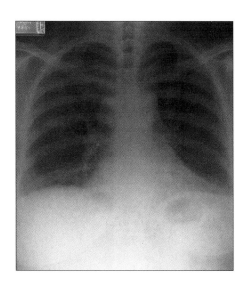

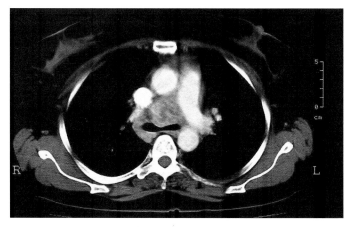

▲ 123

This young woman was treated with rifampicin, isoniazid and pyrazinamide for a tuberculous neck gland. The chest X-ray (upper) was taken before therapy started, and the CT scan (lower) 2 months later.

a) What changes have occurred?

b) Are any changes in therapy indicated?

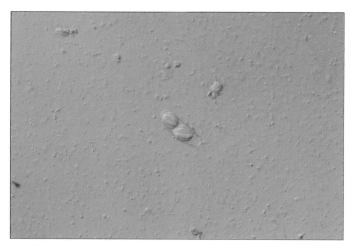

▲ 124

This is a high power view (Nomarski phase microscopy) of a fecal smear from a patient with AIDS who developed watery diarrhea after a short holiday in Africa.
a) What does it show?
b) How should he be treated?

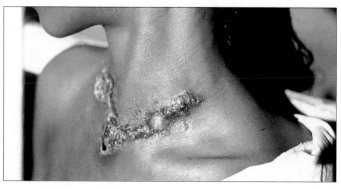

▲ 125

This young woman had lived in the Sudan. The lesion shown had been present for several months.
What is it?

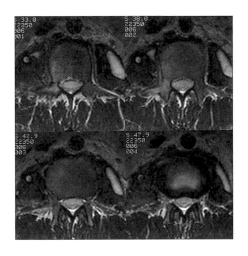

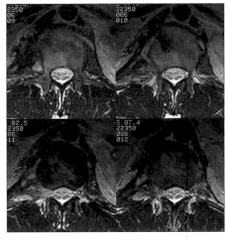

▲ 126

The patient was a young man who had complained of back pain for 1 year.

a) What is shown on the magnetic resonance scan through the psoas muscles (upper) and the vertebral body (lower)?

b) What is the likely primary site of infection?

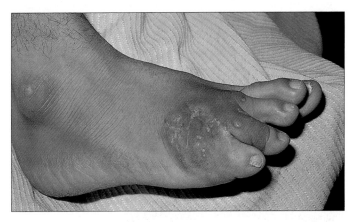

▲ 127

The abnormality shown had developed slowly over about 10 years and was not painful.
a) What is the diagnosis?
b) How would you establish the etiology?

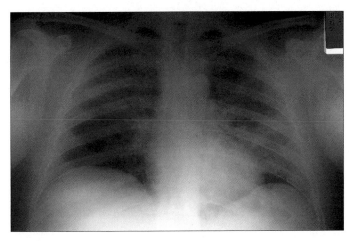

▲ 128

The chest X-ray was taken 6 hours after an expatriate was given quinine for acute falciparum malaria.
What is the etiology of the lesion shown?

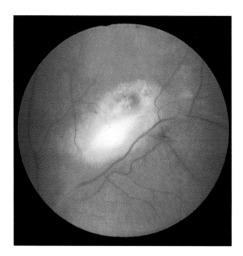

◄ 129

A young man presented with painless loss of vision in his eye 6 months after working on an Australian sheep farm.

a) What is the diagnosis?
b) How should he be treated?

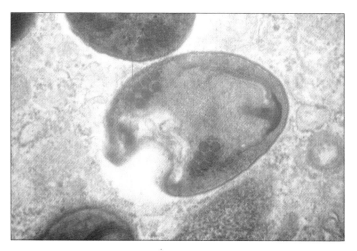

▲ 130

This electron micrograph shows an object approximately 1.5 μm in length, in the feces of a patient with profuse diarrhea and AIDS.

a) What is it?
b) What specific treatment is available?

131 ▶

An intravenous drug user with HIV infection had suffered from recurrent painful vulval lesions for more than 1 month.

a) How can these lesions be prevented?
b) Do they have any other diagnostic implications?

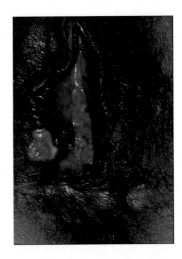

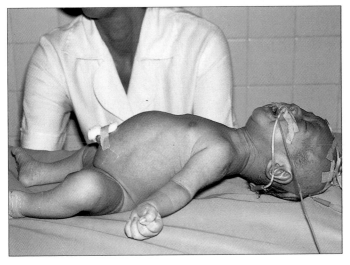

▲ **132**

This neonate became ill with feeding difficulties.

a) What is the cause of the infant's illness?
b) Where is the likely focus of infection?

(See Acknowledgements)

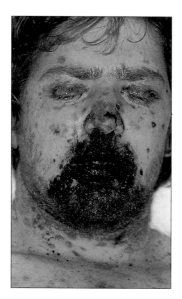

This man has dysuria and a rash on his genitalia, trunk and the soles of his feet, in addition to the lesions illustrated.

a) What is the diagnosis?
b) What infections may be responsible for this condition?

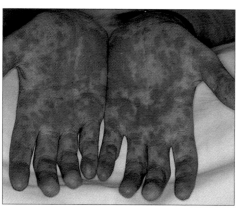

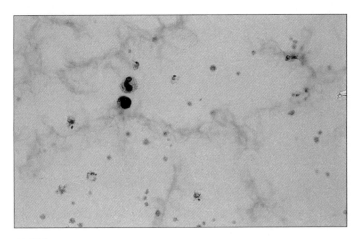

▲ 134
The figure shows a high power view of a blood film taken from a young Indian man who developed fever after an otherwise uncomplicated appendectomy in Britain. He had last visited India 6 months previously.
a) How has the blood film been prepared?
b) What is the diagnosis?

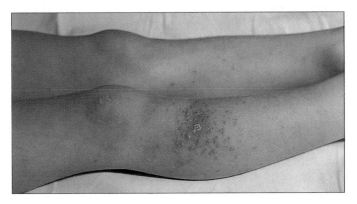

▲ 135
The patient had a sparse, generalized vesicular rash and also complained of a recent boil on the right leg.
What is the diagnosis?

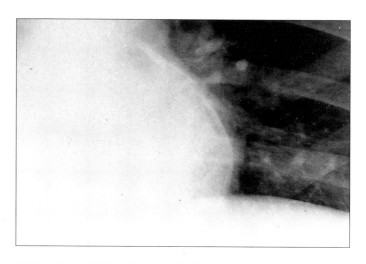

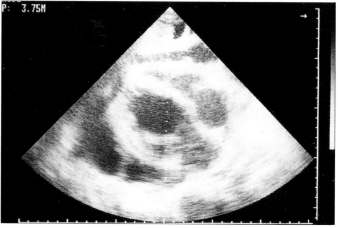

▲ 136

Both these patients presented with limited exercise tolerance. The chest X-ray (upper) is from a 55-year-old British man, and the transthoracic echocardiogram (lower) is from a 25-year-old Malawian man.

a) What abnormality is present in each figure?
b) What diagnosis is common to both patients?
c) What other condition(s) would you exclude?

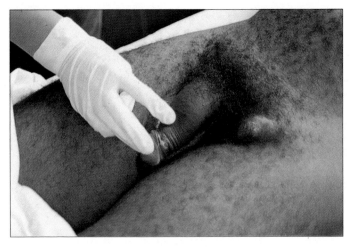

▲ 137

This sailor had recently arrived from West Africa.
a) What physical signs are present?
b) What are the possible diagnoses?

138 ▶

The patient was receiving
intensive chemotherapy for a
non-Hodgkin's lymphoma.
a) What intercurrent infection
   is present?
b) What complications may
   follow?
c) How should the infection be
   treated?

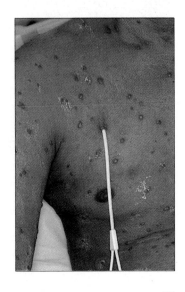

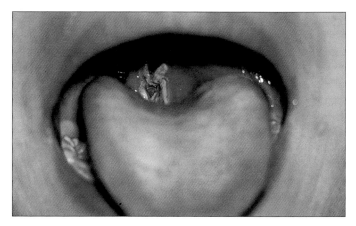

▲ 139

The patient had been traveling in Pakistan for 2 months.

a) What is the cause of the pharyngitis?
b) What immediate treatment is necessary?
c) How is the diagnosis confirmed?

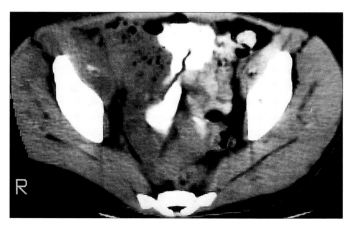

▲ 140

The contrast enhanced CT scan was taken because of difficulty walking. The patient routinely injected drugs into both groins.

a) What abnormalities are present?
b) What physical sign is usually present?

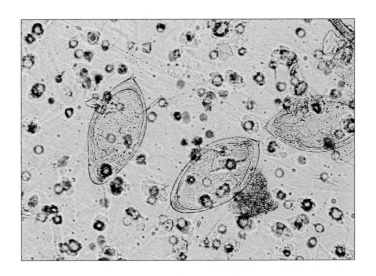

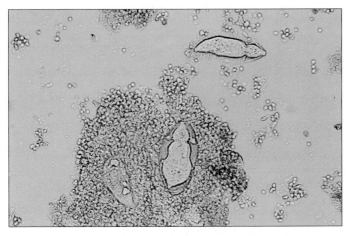

▲ 141

A young man had vague discomfort on ejaculation. He had swum in Lake Malawi 4 months previously. The upper figure shows an unstained nucleopore filter of his urine, and the lower shows an unstained wet preparation of his ejaculate (both high power views).

What is the diagnosis?

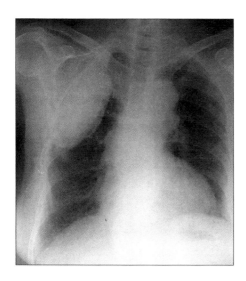

◀ **142**
What does this archival chest X-ray show?

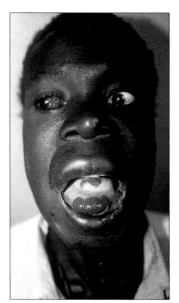

◀ **143**
What are the diagnoses?

144 ▶

This patient had been visiting a fruit farm in South Africa.

a) What is the likely cause of this patient's illness?

b) What is the causative organism?

c) How is it spread?

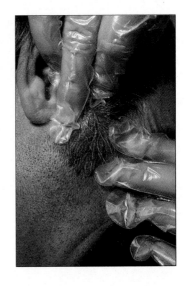

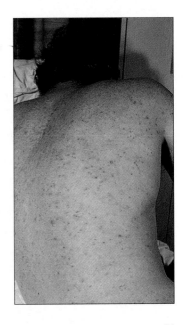

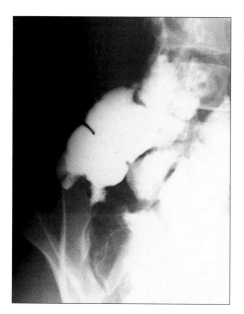

This Saudi male had
abdominal pain and
vague swelling in
his right iliac fossa.
What do the barium
enema views show?

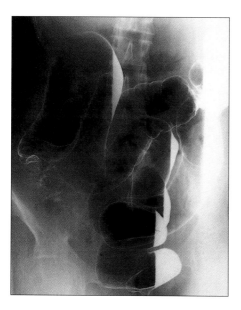

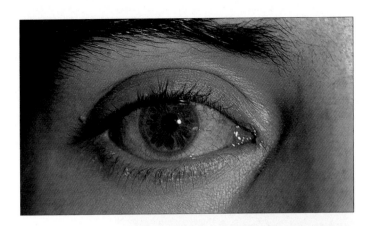

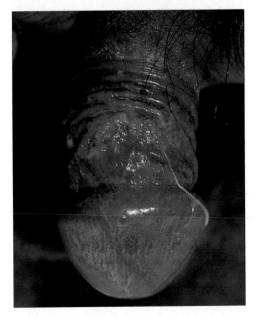

▲ 146

This patient developed polyarthritis associated with dysuria.

a) What is the diagnosis?

b) What is the infective cause?

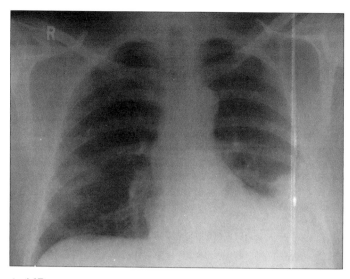

▲ 147
The patient had a persistent cough. The radiological findings were unaltered over a period of 6 weeks.
What points in the medical history are relevant?

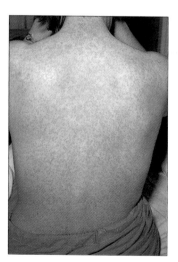

◀ 148
This young woman complained of general malaise of a few days' duration. She had missed a period.
What action is necessary?

149 ▶

The blood film was obtained from a patient who had been treated 3 weeks previously for "malaria" after a prolonged safari in Uganda, where he had received many insect bites.

a) What does it show?

b) What treatment is indicated?

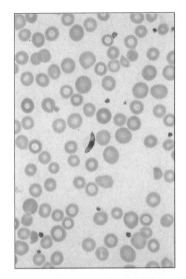

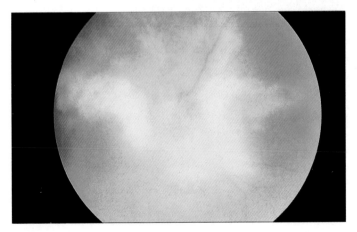

▲ 150

This patient with AIDS had been receiving regular ganciclovir for CMV retinitis, and the photograph was taken after his vision suddenly worsened.

a) What complication has arisen?

b) What is the prognosis for the eye?

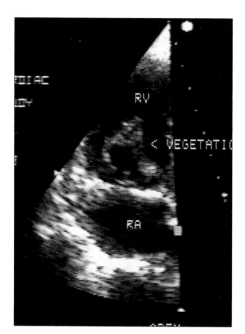

◀ 151
This young woman has a large vegetation attached to the tricuspid valve (transthoracic echocardiogram). What factors predispose to this?

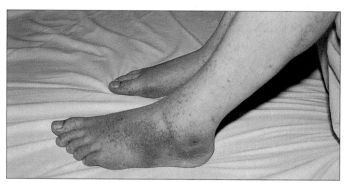

▲ 152
The lesions illustrated developed after treatment with α-interferon for chronic active hepatitis and chronic glomerulonephritis, secondary to hepatitis B carriage. The patient was a hemophiliac and was also anti-HCV antibody positive.
What is the cause?

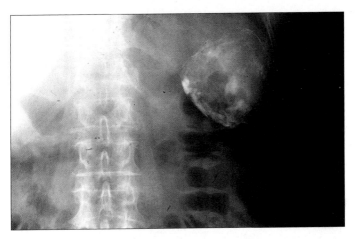

▲ 153

The X-ray was taken after an elderly Maori presented with short-lived diarrhea.

a) What abnormality is shown and what is the differential diagnosis?

b) What treatment is indicated?

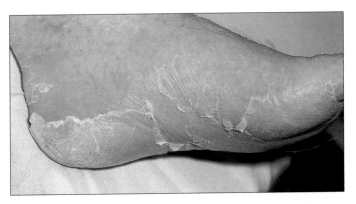

▲ 154

The photograph was taken 2 weeks after the patient presented with shock, jaundice and adult respiratory distress syndrome.

a) What does it show?

b) What are the likely infective causes?

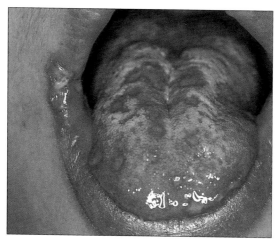

▲ 155

This young woman had difficulty eating.
a) What is the diagnosis?
b) How would you confirm it?
c) How is it treated?

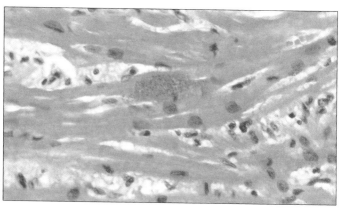

▲ 156

This is a high power view (hematoxylin and eosin) of ventricular tissue from a man who died of fever complicating AIDS.
What is the histological diagnosis?

157 ▶

This 45-year-old man was admitted to hospital with a liver abscess.
a) What abnormalities are present in the chest X-rays?
b) What investigations are indicated?

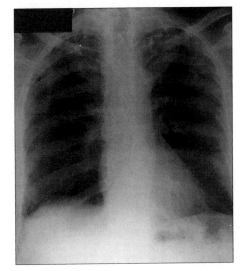

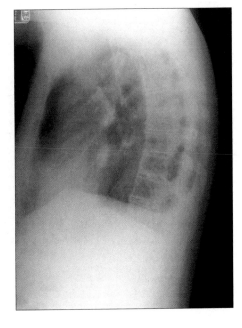

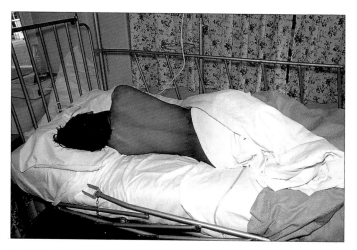

▲ 158
What is the differential diagnosis?

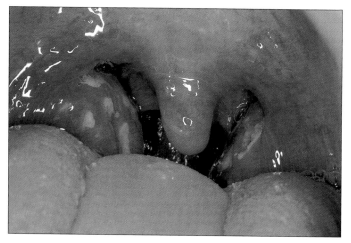

▲ 159
a) What is the likely cause?
b) How might the diagnosis be confirmed?
c) What antibiotic therapy is indicated?

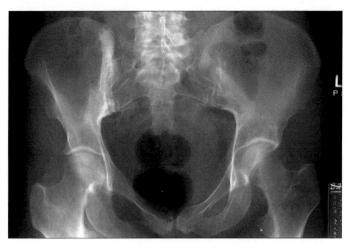

▲ 160

This 55-year-old woman presented with fever. She had a history of recurrent furunculosis. *Staphylococcus aureus* was isolated from multiple blood cultures.

What was the focus of her infection?

161 ▶

The patient presented with fever, vomiting and a skin rash.

a) What clinical condition is shown?

b) What is its natural history?

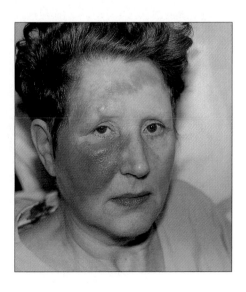

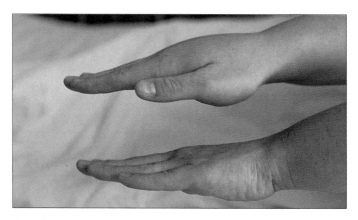

▲ 162

This expatriate, living in Nigeria, developed transient swellings on his hand and had marked peripheral blood eosinophilia.

a) What is this condition called?

b) What causes it?

c) How should it be treated?

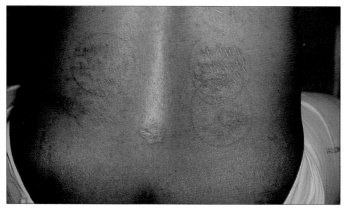

▲ 163

This man from the Middle East had a long history of back pain and occasional fever.

a) What infectious diagnoses should be considered?

b) What lesions are visible?

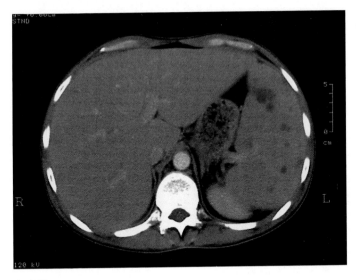

▲ 164

A 38-year-old man with AIDS developed high swinging fever, diarrhea and abdominal pain.

a) What does the CT scan show?

b) How could the diagnosis be confirmed?

165 ▶

The jejunal biopsy illustrated (hematoxylin and eosin) was taken from a West Indian immigrant who had abdominal pain, chronic diarrhea and eosinophilia.

a) What does it show?

b) How should it be treated?

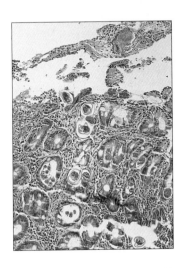

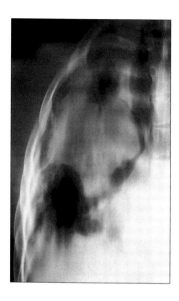

◄ 166
The tomogram illustrated was taken after the patient developed profuse hemoptysis.
a) What is the diagnosis?
b) What is the treatment?

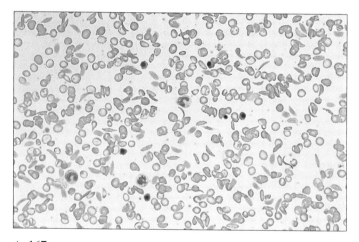

▲ 167
The blood film illustrated was taken from a young West Indian man who presented with jaundice and shock.
a) What is demonstrated?
b) What is the likely infection?

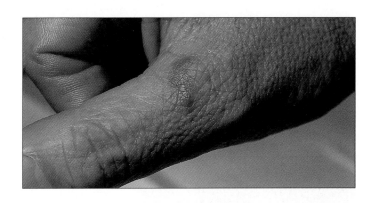

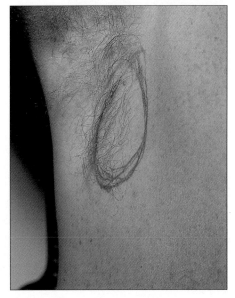

▲ 168
A vet presented with pain and swelling in his right axilla which had developed over 15 days.
a) What is the likely diagnosis?
b) What organism is responsible?
c) What treatment is indicated?

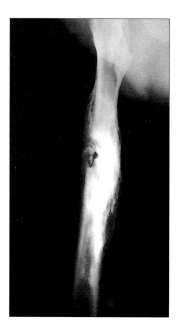

◄ 169

a) What is shown on this plain radiograph of a femur?

b) What long term systemic complication may be associated with this infection?

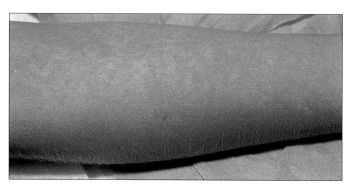

▲ 170

This young woman had just returned from a holiday in Thailand and presented with headache, fever, a rash and mild disturbance of liver function tests and thrombocytopenia.

a) What diagnosis would you consider?

b) What is the prognosis?

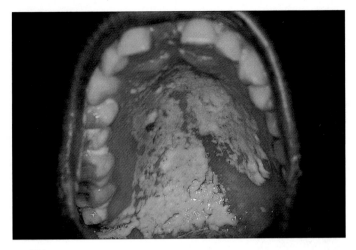

▲ **171**
a) What condition is illustrated?
b) How may it be treated?

172 ▶
This young woman developed a "boil" in the natal cleft while on holiday in Zimbabwe. Petroleum jelly has been applied.
a) What is the diagnosis?
b) How can it be avoided?

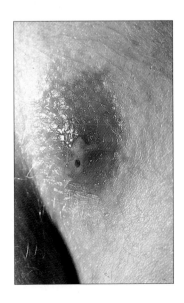

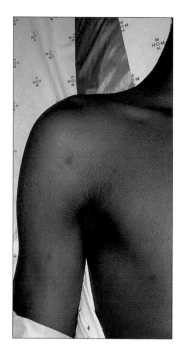

◀ 173

This young man presented with fever and headache and his CSF suggested pyogenic meningitis with no organisms seen on Gram stain. He was not immunosuppressed.

a) What is the probable diagnosis?
b) The rash illustrated is not always so visible. How else would you detect it?

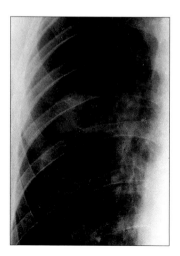

◀ 174

A man with late stage AIDS and neutropenia presented with fever, dysuria and right-sided chest pain.

a) What does the chest X-ray show?
b) What are the likely pathogens?

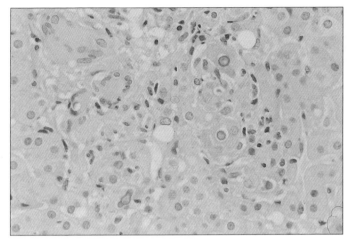

▲ 175

A man with AIDS developed abdominal pain, fever and moderate disturbance of liver function tests. A high power view of his liver biopsy is illustrated (mucicarmine stain).

a) What is the infecting organism?

b) How should he be treated?

176 ▶

An 86-year-old woman was referred for investigation of ataxia.

a) What does her chest X-ray show?

b) What tests are indicated?

c) Are there any hazards from treatment?

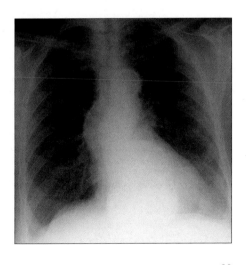

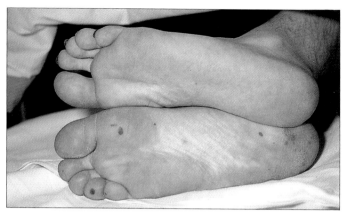

◄ 177

a) What abnormality is present?

b) What is the likely organism?

c) Where has it come from?

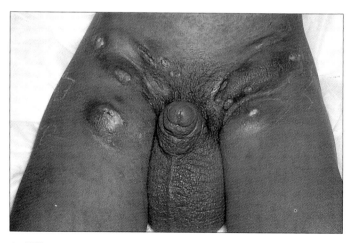

▲ 178

a) What physical signs are present?

b) What diagnoses would you consider?

1 a) He has an epigastric mass and the most likely diagnosis is hepato-cellular carcinoma complicating hepatitis B carriage. Other primary or secondary tumors are possible, and tuberculosis is less likely.

b) There was a bruit over the epigastric mass suggesting hepatocellular carcinoma. He was HBsAg positive and serum α-fetoprotein was markedly elevated. Ultrasonography suggested a hepatoma and liver biopsy was not considered necessary.

c) The prognosis is dismal. He died 1 month later.

2 a) The commonest causative organisms are *Staphylococcus aureus* and β-hemolytic streptococci. The organism in this case was a group G streptococcus.

b) Blood cultures. Antistreptolysin "O" titers. An attempt may be made to isolate the organism by injecting a little sterile saline into the skin and culturing the aspirate.

c) She is at risk of bacteremic spread of infection to the hip prosthesis.

3 a) Cutaneous leishmaniasis or cutaneous tuberculosis are the most likely diagnoses.

b) Biopsy showed non-caseating granulomata containing very scanty amastigotes of a *Leishmania* sp. These failed to grow on appropriate media (NNN). Leishmania serology was negative.

4 a) The biopsy shows the pear shaped trophozoites of *Giardia lamblia* in the bowel lumen.

b) Cyst excretion is intermittent, and microscopy of further fecal specimens is sometimes necessary to make the diagnosis. Upper intestinal fluid sampling by string test is at least as sensitive as jejunal biopsy in difficult cases.

5 a) There is destruction of the L5/S1 disc with involvement of the body of the vertebrae on either side of the disc. The appearance is typical of tuberculous discitis and osteomyelitis, but other pathogens, especially *Staphylococcus aureus* and *Pseudomonas* sp., should be considered.

b) CT guided aspiration or open biopsy is essential to provide material for mycobacterial and routine culture (TB was confirmed).

6 a) He has cholera.

b) Microscopy of feces for the "shooting star" appearance of motile *Vibrio cholerae*, confirmed by neutralization of motility by specific antisera. Culture of feces.

7 a) The patient has psoriasis, the satellite lesions also suggesting a fungal infection.

b) This man has moderately advanced HIV infection, with exacerb-ation of psoriasis as a presenting feature.

8 a) This section shows replacement of normal liver architecture by bands of fibrosis with inflammatory cells at the margins, separating nodules of hepatocytes. Proliferating bile ductules are seen within the fibrous tissue.

  b) This is established cirrhosis which could be due to hepatitis B and/or hepatitis C.

9 a) Palatal petechiae.

  b) Infectious mononucleosis and rubella.

10 a) The most likely diagnosis is pulmonary hydatid cyst due to *Echinococcus granulosus*. Other possibilities include metastases from tumors, especially seminomas, or a tumor arising from the chest wall.

  b) Dogs are the usual primary hosts in Wales, with cysts found in herbivores such as sheep and cattle.

  c) The cyst may remain asymptomatic. If it ruptures the patient is likely to present with hemoptysis and may expectorate cyst material, sometimes associated with wheeze or anaphylaxis.

11 There is a marked local sensitivity reaction to tetanus toxoid: antibiotic treatment is not indicated. Most patients who experience such reactions have adequate humoral immunity to tetanus and should not be given further doses of toxoid.

12 Epstein-Barr virus, cytomegalovirus, varicella zoster, human immunodeficiency virus, *Borrelia burgdorferi*. The patient has a facial palsy.

13 a) He has destruction of the nasal bones due to endemic syphilis (bejel) acquired in childhood. The associated hard palate lesion could also be caused by congenital syphilis, and makes the other differential diagnoses of leprosy, tuberculosis or leishmaniasis unlikely.

  b) He had weakly positive reaginic (VDRL) and specific (FTA, TPHA) tests for syphilis.

14 a) There is invasion through the wall of the blood vessel by a cluster of organisms with a yeast-like appearance where they are seen in the blood vessel lumen. This is the appearance of disseminated candidiasis.

  b) Silver based stains such as Grocott's stain, or PAS stain, will demonstrate most fungal pathogens.

15 *Herpes simplex* virus. Herpetic whitlow may be acquired by contact with saliva containing the causative organism, for example during nursing procedures. The lesions should be treated with an oral antiviral such as acyclovir.

16 a) Both maxillary antra contain fluid levels.

  b) Culture of aspirate from the sinuses yielded *Streptococcus pneumoniae*. Patients with HIV are also at increased risk of *Pseudomonas aeruginosa* and fungal infections of the sinuses, although the latter would be less likely to produce such marked fluid levels.

17 a) It is the fish tapeworm *Diphyllobothrium latum.*

b) This is usually acquired by eating inadequately cooked or raw fish (especially in Finland).

c) Infected individuals are usually asymptomatic or, as in this case, notice intermittent passage of motile tapeworm segments per rectum. The large adult tapeworm competes selectively for vitamin B12 and may cause anemia.

18 a) A vascular lesion has developed at the site of a venepuncture.

b) Behçets disease. Her symptoms were controlled with low dose colchicine.

19 Typhoid fever. The typical "rose spots" on the abdomen contain the causative organism.

20 Chickenpox pneumonia is commoner or more severe in adults, smokers, the immunodeficient and during pregnancy.

21 a) The patient has cytomegalovirus (CMV) retinitis. There are destructive hemorrhagic retinal lesions distributed along blood vessels.

b) Diagnosis is based on clinical appearances coupled with a response to therapy with ganciclovir or phosphonoformate.

c) CMV may also cause neuropathy, polyradiculitis, encephalopathy, pneumonitis, hepatitis, cholecystitis, colitis and adrenalitis.

22 a) Pneumococcal septicemia following splenectomy. Splenectomy also predisposes to infection with *Neisseria meningitidis* and *Haemophilus influenzae* type B.

b) Pneumococcal vaccination, which should be repeated after five years. There is also an option for giving additional long-term prophylaxis with oral penicillin. Some authorities advocate meningococcal and *H. influenzae* vaccination.

23 a) Both men had suffered painless burns from the hot water pipe behind their legs. They both have scars of previous injuries.

b) Peripheral sensory neuropathy due to leprosy. Neither was diabetic.

c) Both had palpable thickening of several nerves and one patient had pronounced neuropathic changes in his hands.

24 a) There are multiple lesions of florid scabies.

b) He was not HIV positive. Biopsy of an enlarged lymph node confirmed non-Hodgkin's lymphoma.

25 a) The most likely diagnosis is aphthous ulcers, but syphilis, herpes simplex and CMV infections should be excluded. The larger central lesion has overlying candidiasis. Biopsy may be necessary for solitary lesions to exclude lymphoma or invasive fungal infection.

b) Empirical acyclovir failed, as did antiseptic mouthwashes. The lesions responded dramatically to thalidomide.

26 a) There is a lytic lesion in the tarsal bones, with gas extending from the sole of the foot up to the top of the calf.

b) The patient has chronic osteomyelitis with secondary anaerobic infection. He is a diabetic.

27 Negative pressure containment isolators may be used for the transport of patients with suspected or proven viral hemorrhagic fevers (Lassa, Marburg, Ebola and Crimean-Congo).

28 a) A chickenpox rash may be more difficult to diagnose on black skins. However this eruption is typical in the way it is concentrated in anatomical concavities.

b) Electron microscopy of vesicle fluid will reveal typical herpes particles.

29 a) Poliomyelitis.

b) Physiotherapy and splinting in the acute stage help to prevent the development of flexion contractures.

30 Maxillary and palatal herpes zoster, with left sided lower motor neuron facial palsy.

31 a) The GP asked for early morning specimens of urine to be examined for tubercle bacilli.

b) The Ziehl-Neelsen stained smear shows scanty acid alcohol-fast bacilli. The patient had a tuberculous ureteric stricture, hydroureter, and secondary bacterial urinary infections.

32 a) There is exaggeration of the cortical sulci, out of keeping with the patient's age, suggesting cortical atrophy.

b) A full "dementia screen" is required and HIV testing is essential. This patient had HIV-related dementia.

c) Some patients respond well to relatively high doses of zidovudine.

33 a) The lower pole of the cecum and the ileocecal junction have a ragged appearance.

b) Such an appearance could be due to Crohn's disease, tuberculosis or yersiniosis but the most likely cause in this man is cytomegalovirus.

c) Examination of the optic fundi showed bilateral active CMV retinitis.

34 a) Falciparum malaria (*Plasmodium falciparum*).

b) The film illustrated shows several erythrocytes containing more than one parasite. All the parasites present are early trophozoite ring forms, more than 1% of the erythrocytes are infected and some of the parasites adhere to the inside of the erythrocyte membrane. This film does not contain a characteristic gametocyte.

35 a) Herpes zoster induced iritis and keratitis.

b) There is involvement of the nasociliary nerve with lesions on the nose. 50% of patients with nasociliary nerve involvement will develop eye complications.

36 a) Fever, headache and a rash might suggest typhoid, meningococcal disease or arbovirus infection but the rashes are not typical. Both men had unprotected sex in Thailand and the first patient (upper) had an HIV seroconversion illness. The second had secondary syphilis.

b) Anti-HIV antibody ELISA on serum from the first patient (upper) was negative at presentation, but became positive 2 months later. His serum p24 levels were raised. His syphilis serology was negative. The second patient had negative HIV antibody tests for 1 year after presentation but had strongly positive serum VDRL and TPHA tests.

37 a) There is a large lower lobe lung abscess.

b) Common pathogens include *Staphylococcus aureus*, *Streptococcus milleri*, *Klebsiella aerogenes* and anaerobes (*Bacteroides* spp.). Infection is often polymicrobial.

38 a) Cutaneous larva migrans due to larvae of dog or cat hookworms.

b) Topical application of thiabendazole, or oral albendazole or ivermectin. Oral thiabendazole could be used but has more side effects.

39 a) Pertussis (whooping cough)

b) Severe periorbital bruising caused by high venous pressure in the superior vena cava during paroxysms of coughing.

40 Hemorrhagic chickenpox. A rare bleeding diathesis in which either immune thrombocytopenia or disseminated intravascular coagulation may play a part.

41 a) Anthrax.

b) A Gram stained smear of material taken from the lesion will reveal the Gram positive rods of *Bacillus anthracis*.

42 a) There are three hemorrhages and a single soft exudate associated with blood vessels. The pigmentation of the fundus is normal for a woman of African origin.

b) The most likely diagnosis is Roth's spots, associated with endocarditis. Alternatives include systemic lupus erythematosus, or CMV complicating HIV infection.

c) With the short history and florid lesions, *Staphylococcus aureus* is the most likely pathogen and was present in all her blood cultures.

43 a) A man of this age is more likely to have an obstructive cause for jaundice, including gallstones and primary and secondary tumors, or a drug-induced hepatitis. Chronic hepatitis due to hepatitis B or C is unlikely to cause this much jaundice unless he has decompensated liver failure or has a complicating hepatoma. Hepatitis A is very unlikely due to his age. Leptospirosis was excluded. He had acute hepatitis E.

b) Ultrasonography of the liver, biliary tree and pancreas to exclude obstructive lesions. Prothrombin time and serum albumin for initial assessment of liver function.

44 a) The patient had acute herpes simplex encephalitis. The magnetic resonance scan shows extensive necrosis of the left temporal lobe.

b) For diagnosis, examination of the CSF for specific antibody and for viral DNA (by polymerase chain reaction) is preferable to more hazardous brain biopsy.

c) Two weeks' treatment with high dose intravenous acyclovir reduces morbidity and mortality. It should be started as soon as the diagnosis is suspected.

45 Opportunistic infections including candidiasis, cryptococcosis, histoplasmosis and with *Pneumocystis carinii* may present with skin involvement. Lymphoma and atypical Kaposi's sarcoma are also strong possibilities. In this case biopsy revealed non-Hodgkin's lymphoma.

46 Herpangina. The characteristic papules and ulcers are concentrated in the pharynx and the back of the mouth. Coxsackie A viruses are the usual causes.

47 a) Tinea pedis, caused by *Trichophyton rubrum* or *T. mentagrophytes.*

b) Microscopy and culture (Sabouraud's agar) of skin scrapings. Topical imidazole treatment, for example clotrimazole cream or powder, is usually effective.

48 a) The colon is grossly dilated.

b) The patient had a toxic megacolon associated with salmonella infection. Other possible causes include acute inflammatory bowel disease, amebic colitis and pseudomembranous colitis.

49 a) The distended veins suggest femoral vein occlusion. Erythema and swelling above the inguinal ligament suggest infection (abscess, septic thrombophlebitis, or both).

b) He has a 50% chance of having bacteremia and blood cultures are essential. Other investigations for endocarditis including echocardiography might be considered. Venous occlusion should be investigated by venography or MR scan.

50 Apart from malignant transformation of his tumor, superimposed tuberculosis must be ruled out. Biopsy of one of the glands showed acid fast bacilli, cultured as *Mycobacterium tuberculosis.*

51 a) There is a collection of pale histiocytes with a central microabscess containing neutrophils and cellular debris. This is pseudotuberculosis due to infection with *Yersinia* sp.

b) Cotrimoxazole, doxycycline or ciprofloxacin by mouth, or systemic gentamicin in septicemic infections.

52 a) Ascending polyneuritis (Guillain-Barré syndrome).

b) A link to recent *Campylobacter jejuni* infections has been suggested. CMV, HIV and occasionally coxsackievirus or echoviruses have also been associated with the syndrome.

c) Intubation and mechanical ventilation. Steroids alone are no more effective than placebo. Plasma exchange and high dose intravenous immunoglobulins both have demonstrated benefit.

53 a) There are calcified cysts in the cervical and occipital muscles and in the chest wall.

b) The pig tapeworm, *Taenia solium*.

c) Praziquantel or albendazole. Patients are usually given adjunctive steroids during the initial phase of chemotherapy, to reduce reactive edema around intracranial cysts.

54 a) Pyoderma gangrenosum.

b) He developed ulcerative colitis. Pyoderma gangrenosum may be associated with (or precede) inflammatory bowel disease or rheumatoid arthritis.

55 a) Any septicemia, but the lesions and history suggest disseminated candidiasis.

b) Systemic antifungal therapy with amphotericin B, or an imidazole such as fluconazole, should be started immediately after several sets of blood cultures and skin biopsy.

56 a) Cutaneous leishmaniasis, due to *Leishmania tropica*.

b) Dissemination of cutaneous leishmaniasis acquired in the Indian subcontinent in unusual, and specific antileishmanial treatment is not always indicated. Topical paromomycin cream may be as effective as systemic antimonials.

57 a) The liver biopsy contains two non-caseating granulomas, more suggestive of brucellosis than of tuberculosis. The differential is large.

b) Blood cultures and serology for brucellosis (and Q fever), culture of the liver biopsy material for *Brucella* sp. and *Mycobacterium tuberculosis*.

58 a) The usual cause of napkin rash is simple (chemical) contact dermatitis. This child has satellite lesions suggesting superimposed candidiasis.

b) Exposure to the air and an emollient skin cream. Suspected or proven candidal infection can be treated with a topical agent such as clotrimazole.

59 a) This combination of symptoms strongly suggests a diagnosis of cryptococcal meningitis, and the fundus shows exudative lesions in addition to papilledema.

b) After CT brain scan to exclude a space occupying lesion, CSF should be examined for cryptococci by India ink stain, assay for cryptococcal antigen and culture.

60 a) Infectious diagnoses to consider included histoplasmoma, cocci-dioidomycosis, aspergilloma (usually cavitating), tuberculoma and *Dirofilaria immitis* (the dog heartworm).

b) She had not lived in a coccidioidomycosis or histoplasmosis endemic area or visited caves, and she had no exposure to dogs. There was no family or personal history of known TB. This was a histoplasmoma.

61 a) Florid petechial rash and neck retraction.

b) Meningococcal meningitis.

c) Parenteral antibiotics. Penicillin would almost certainly be appropriate, but other pathogens can occasionally produce a similar syndrome and we would treat with a third generation cephalosporin until there was laboratory confirmation of meningococcal disease.

62 a) Roundworms (*Ascaris lumbricoides*). The feces should be examined microscopically for ova of other helminths, particularly hookworm and *Trichuris trichura*, which frequently are also present in this setting.

b) A broad spectrum anthelmintic such as mebendazole or albendazole would be appropriate.

63 a) Infectious mononucleosis

b) T-lymphocytes, mounting an immune response to Epstein-Barr virus infected B lymphocytes.

64 Hepatitis B carriage may be associated with polyarteritis nodosa.

65 a) Herpes zoster: reactivated varicella-zoster virus infection.

b) Zoster in children characteristically follows primary varicella infection which has occurred very early in life, either *in utero* or in infancy.

66 Infectious mononucleosis. The illness is occasionally accompanied by a short-lived erythematous macular rash. More florid rashes are usually associated with drug reactions to semi-synthetic penicillins, particularly ampicillin and amoxycillin.

67 a) The knee X-ray shows total disruption of the normal anatomy. The pelvic X-ray shows numerous round shadows in both gluteal areas.

b) She has tabes dorsalis, with Charcot's joints secondary to the sensory neuropathy. The ring shadows represent bismuth injections given as treatment in the pre-penicillin era for syphilis.

68 a) He is jaundiced with bruising and bleeding at the sites of vene-puncture and IV line insertion.

b) Severe leptospirosis (Weil's disease). With the history of water contact, the most likely species is *Leptospira icterohemorrhagiae*.

69 a) It shows typical features of a fungal infection, with non-branching pseudo-hyphae stained black. In this context, candidal esophagitis is the diagnosis.

b) This patient was HIV positive and this was his AIDS-defining illness. *Candida* esophagitis may also complicate the treatment of hematological malignancies or lymphomas, and only occasionally occurs in immunocompetent patients.

70 a) The skin biopsy (Fite's method, equivalent to Ziehl-Neelsen) is packed with acid fast bacilli. She has multibacillary leprosy.

b) Nasal smear confirmed that she was excreting *Mycobacterium leprae*. Although infectious to others, the risk of transmission is relatively low.

71 a) Fournier's gangrene is a form of necrotizing fasciitis that characteristically affects the scrotal region.

b) A wide range of organisms, both aerobic and anaerobic, may be responsible.

c) Widespread excision should be combined with broad spectrum antimicrobial therapy, such as clindamycin plus an aminoglycoside. The benefit of hyperbaric oxygen therapy is unproven.

72 The scan shows evidence of graft infection. There is gas within the lumen and wall of the aortic graft, spreading laterally into retroperitoneal tissues. Part of the graft lumen is occluded by thrombus. *Streptococcus milleri* and *Bacteroides fragilis* were isolated from blood cultures.

73 a) The diagnosis was scabies. The skin biopsy revealed an acarus of *Sarcoptes scabei* lying in a typical burrow.

b) Treatment is with whole-body applications of lindane, malathion or permethrin. Lindane must be avoided in pregnancy and lactation.

74 Bubonic plague. Aspiration of fluid from the bubo for staining by either Gram's or Wayson's methods, and culture for *Yersinia pestis*.

75 Hand-foot-and-mouth disease. Various enteroviruses, usually coxsackie A16 or some echoviruses, are responsible.

76 Tuberculous meningitis. There is streaky right upper lobe shadowing on the chest X-ray. Mycobacterium tuberculosis was isolated from sputum and CSF.

77 This is an archival photograph showing eczema vaccinatum acquired from a relative who had recently been vaccinated against smallpox. Other virus infections causing similar appearances include herpes simplex (eczema herpeticum) and molluscum contagiosum.

78 a) The upper CT scan shows an infected and fluid filled right maxillary sinus. The ethmoid sinus is also infected.

b) The lower two scans shows a dilated ventricular system consistent with communicating hydrocephalus.

79 a) There is a pyopneumothorax together with an intrapulmonary fluid level on the left, and a small peripheral lung abscess in the lateral right lower zone.

b) The radiographic appearance is of multiple lung abscesses, one of which has ruptured to produce the pyopneumothorax. The most common cause is hematogenous dissemination of *Staphylococcus aureus* from peripheral abscesses or IV lines, or as in this case, from right sided endocarditis secondary to drug abuse.

80 a) Kaposi's sarcoma
   b) Steroids and antibiotics to control the swelling and secondary infection.

81 Extensive pelvic sepsis. There is gas in the soft tissues implying infection with *Clostridium spp.* and other gas forming anaerobes.

82 a) There is pigmented chorioretinitis, which is typical of old ocular toxoplasmosis.
   b) Low titers of IgG anti-toxoplasma antibodies would suggest the diagnosis.
   c) At this stage, probably none. Recurrence of symptoms due to reactivation would require active chemotherapy.

83 a) Trachoma. Extensive inflammatory nodules are visible on the palpebral conjunctiva.
   b) *Chlamydia trachomatis.*
   c) Topical tetracycline is of marginal benefit. Systemic antibiotics would eradicate the organism but scarring is likely to persist in such advanced disease.

84 a) There are poorly defined infiltrates in both lung fields. Many causes need to be considered, including Kaposi's sarcoma, *Mycobacterium tuberculosis* and *Mycobacterium avium complex*, CMV, *Pneumocystis carinii*, aspergillosis and cryptococcosis.
   b) Microscopy (with appropriate stains) and culture of induced sputum. Bronchoscopy with bronchoalveolar lavage and transbronchial biopsy.

85 a) This is post-dysenteric Reiter's syndrome, a type of reactive arthritis caused by *Salmonella* spp., *Shigella* spp., *Campylobacter jejuni* and *Yersinia enterocolitica*. Diarrhea may also complicate Reiter's syndrome associated with non-gonococcal urethritis.
   b) Possession of the HLA B27 phenotype.

86 Measles. In the prodromal stages the characteristic Koplik's spots may be found on the buccal mucosa.

87 a) Severe Stevens-Johnson syndrome, in this context suggestive of HIV infection.
   b) The most likely culprit in this case is thiacetazone, but rifampicin has also been implicated. Ingestion of other drugs such as sulfur-containing compounds should be excluded.

88 a) Filoviridae are characteristically long thread-like viruses often with curved or crook-like ends.
   b) Marburg and Ebola viral hemorrhagic fevers.

89 a) The biopsy shows extensive central caseation.

   b) Tuberculosis. This was confirmed by culture of the biopsy material.

90 a) Extensive bilateral renal staghorn calculi.

   b) As in this patient, chronic urine infection with *Proteus* sp. particularly predisposes to staghorn calculi, due to struvite deposition secondary to urease production.

91 a) Both feet show the effects of chronic lymphatic obstruction due to filariasis. Similar changes may be seen with non-filarial obstruction in the tropics (podoconiosis), or be associated with congenital lymphatic disorders such as Milroy's disease or surgical damage to lymphatic drainage proximally.

   b) He had recurrent streptococcal infections of his legs despite prophylactic penicillin therapy, and *Streptococcus pyogenes* was present in his blood cultures.

92 Mumps parotitis followed by mumps meningoencephalitis.

93 a) Penicillin-resistant pneumococcal pneumonia or an atypical pneumonia including Legionnaire's disease and Q fever.

   b) Blood and sputum cultures, examination of sputum for pneumococcal antigen, examination of urine for *Legionella* antigen, acute and convalescent serology.

94 a) Erythema nodosum.

   b) An invasive bacterial gut pathogen. Erythema nodosum may follow infection with *Salmonella* spp., *Shigella* spp., *Campylobacter jejuni* or *Yersinia enterocolitica*. It may also occur in association with inflammatory bowel disease.

95 a) *Staphylococcus aureus* phage group II.

   b) Toxic epidermal necrolysis, Lyell's syndrome or "scalded skin syndrome".

   c) The skin damage is mediated by bacterial exotoxins.

96 a) Orf – a pox virus acquired from sheep and goats.

   b) Tissue culture and electron microscopy of material taken from the lesions.

   c) None

97 a) The X-rays show pleural reaction at the right base and an elevated right hemi-diaphragm.

   b) Liver abscess, probably amebic.

   c) Full blood count, blood culture, liver ultrasound, amebic serology.

98 a) Henoch-Shönlein purpura.

   b) May follow streptococcal pharyngitis. Usually no infective trigger is identified.

   c) Intussusception, gastrointestinal bleeding, arthropathy and renal failure.

99 a) Herpes zoster of the C5 dermatome.

b) Post herpetic neuralgia. Motor weakness from involvement of anterior spinal nerve roots is common following herpes zoster involving the upper limbs.

100 Either measles, or a viral upper respiratory tract infection with an associated drug eruption. The presence of Koplik's spots would establish a diagnosis of measles.

101 a) The urine contains a granular cast together with macrophages and a few red cells, a consequence of post-streptococcal glomerulonephritis.

b) The patient's throat culture yielded a heavy growth of *Streptococcus pyogenes* and his ASOT was significantly elevated.

102 a) There is punctate calcification above the left kidney as well as some costochondral calcification. The CT scan shows a small wedge of calcification in an otherwise atrophic left adrenal.

b) She had Addison's disease, secondary to adrenal destruction by previous tuberculosis.

103 a) The photomicrograph is a medium power view stained with Ziehl–Neelsen stain.

b) The rectal biopsy is packed with clumps of acid-fast bacilli and the most likely diagnosis is infection with *Mycobacterium avium* complex which was confirmed by culture of feces and blood. The fundal lesions could be non-specific exudates of HIV or due to MAC. They disappeared after a month of symptom relief with antimycobacterial treatment.

104 a) The CT scan shows a fluid level with gas in the urinary bladder. The posterior wall of the bladder is irregular and communicates with an irregular mass connected to the bowel.

b) Although bowel cancer communicating with the bladder was confirmed histologically, she denied recent changes in bowel habit. She had noticed a foul smell in her urine and the sensation of passing bubbles on micturition.

105 a) She has scars of previous herpes zoster infection.

b) There is a more than 90% chance that she is HIV antibody positive.

106 a) Ecthyma gangrenosum.

b) *Pseudomonas aeruginosa*.

107 a) *Brugia malayi* (filariasis) with characteristic pink staining sheath and a small gap before the terminal tail nucleus.

b) No immediate treatment was required. After she had finished breast feeding, she was treated with diethylcarbamazine. Ivermectin would now be the treatment of choice.

108 a) He has a liver abscess.

b) Anaerobes, bowel organisms, *Streptococcus milleri* or *Entameba histolytica*.

c) A bowel origin should always be excluded in occult liver abscess.

109 a) Immediate Gram stain and culture of the pus, and blood cultures. X-rays of the leg. Metastatic infection to other bones, joints and heart should be considered (bone isotope scan, echocardiography).

b) Formal surgical exploration and irrigation of the knee joint. Systemic broad spectrum antibiotic therapy, including cover for *Staphylococcus aureus* and Gram negative organisms, pending culture results.

110 The photograph shows phlyctenular conjunctivitis, with nodular inflammation on the bulbar conjunctiva. This is an unusual manifestation of tuberculin hypersensitivity occurring shortly after primary infection with tuberculosis.

111 a) The diagnosis was bacterial endocarditis. *Kingella denitrificans* was isolated from blood cultures.

b) The CT brain scan shows hemorrhage in the left frontal lobe, and an infarct in the left occipital lobe.

112 The patient had a fixed drug eruption caused by antibiotic therapy. In this case the sulfonamide component of co-trimoxazole was probably responsible.

113 a) The smear shows typical Gram negative diplococci of *Neisseria meningitidis* within neutrophils. The patient has meningococcal meningitis.

b) The public health authorities should be informed without delay. Close family and kissing contacts should be offered rifampicin or ciprofloxacin prophylaxis. The patient should also be given 48 hours' rifampicin therapy before discharge to eliminate nasopharyngeal carriage of the organism.

114 a) Numerous irregular filling defects in the liver, suggestive of peliosis hepatis.

b) Patients with peliosis hepatis (sometimes associated with *Bartonella henselae* infection) do not usually have eosinophilia, which suggests a worm or fluke infection. She had acute *Fasciola hepatica* (liver fluke) infection.

c) Contrast enhancement to rule out liver abscess. Microscopy of feces for eggs of *F. hepatica*. Serological tests are suggestive but not very specific for fascioliasis.

115 a) He has cellulitis with ascending lymphangitis.

b) This is most likely to be of streptococcal origin.

116 a) Miliary calcification.

b) The differential diagnosis is prior chickenpox, histoplasmosis or, as in this case, miliary tuberculosis.

117 a) Necrotizing fasciitis with streptococcal toxic shock syndrome (*Streptococcus pyogenes*).

b) High dose parenteral penicillin and aggressive surgical debridement.

118 a) It shows a high intensity signal lesion in the cerebellum. There is also sinusitis on the contralateral side.

b) The main infectious causes are PML (progressive multifocal leuko-encephalopathy) caused by polyomavirus, or toxoplasmosis. At autopsy he had a necrotic B-cell lymphoma of the brain stem and cerebellum.

119 a) He had acute necrotizing gingivostomatitis.

b) A variety of peptostreptococci and Gram negative anaerobes may be the cause, but treatment is directed at anaerobes. He responded to oral metronidazole.

120 a) The bladder wall is calcified. There is also a lesion outside the bladder which could be a large ureteric stone or a phlebolith.

b) Long-standing schistosomiasis. Praziquantel.

121 a) There is swelling and erythema of the bridge of the nose with edema of the eyelids. Although cellulitis is the most common cause, tumor and mucormycosis should be considered.

b) X-rays and CT or MR scans of the facial bones and sinuses, and blood cultures. Mucormycosis often requires aggressive surgery combined with systemic antifungal therapy.

122 a) The patient had chronic pharyngeal candidiasis, with oral and pulmonary Kaposi's sarcoma.

b) AIDS.

123 a) Bihilar lymphadenopathy has developed. Patients with "glandular" tuberculosis often develop reactive lymphadenopathy in the early stages of chemotherapy.

b) No change in the antituberculous regimen is indicated. Patients with symptomatic adenopathy sometimes benefit from a short course of steroids. Her bihilar adenopathy resolved before the end of chemotherapy.

124 a) It shows an oocyst of *Isospora belli*, containing two sporocysts each of which contains four sporozoites.

b) Cotrimoxazole.

125 Scrofuloderma, spread by local implantation of *Mycobacterium tuberculosis* by her necklace.

126 a) The MR scan shows bilateral psoas abscesses, more prominent on the left (upper), and destruction of the vertebral body (lower).

b) He had chronic staphylococcal osteomyelitis of the lower thoracic vertebrae.

127 a) This is a mycetoma (Madura foot) with distortion of tissue and several obvious sinuses.

b) Causative organisms include *Nocardia* spp. and a wide variety of saprophytic fungi. The color of granules discharged from sinuses sometimes suggests the etiological organism, but histological examination and culture of a deep biopsy are preferable.

128 The chest X-ray shows widespread infiltrates. These could be due to adult respiratory distress syndrome due to malaria or concomitant Gram negative septicemia, or to over vigorous fluid replacement therapy.

129 a) Toxocariasis – ocular involvement by the larva of *Toxocara canis*.

b) The patient was given systemic steroids to reduce the edema. Specific antiparasitic therapy is contraindicated, as this may worsen local inflammation and cause further visual loss.

130 a) This is a typical spore of the microsporidian parasite *Enterocytozoon bieneusi*, with two adjacent rows of coiled polar filament seen in cross section near the concave pole (on the left).

b) Unlike *Encephalitozoon* sp. and *Septata intestinalis*, *E. bieneusi* does not respond well to albendazole, the only specific therapy available at the time of writing.

131 a) Recurrent genital herpes can be successfully suppressed by continuous prophylaxis with daily acyclovir.

b) Persistence of herpes simplex for more than a month was her AIDS defining illness.

132 a) The child has opisthotonos, caused by neonatal tetanus.

b) The raw umbilical stump is the usual site of infection of the causative organism, *Clostridium tetani*.

133 a) The Stevens-Johnson syndrome. There is erythema multiforme associated with mucosal lesions of the mouth, eyes, urethra and genitalia.

b) The condition may be triggered by a variety of organisms including *Mycoplasma pneumoniae*, herpes simplex, adenoviruses, coxsackie viruses and streptococcal infections.

134 a) This is a thick blood film, prepared by allowing a blood spot to dry on the slide. Field's stain has been used to stain the slide after washing the unfixed film briefly in tap water. This process destroys the red cells, but leaves white cells, platelets and hemoparasites.

b) The history suggests vivax malaria, and several different stages of *Plasmodium vivax* trophozoites were present in the film.

135 Chickenpox (varicella). The lesions often cluster around the site of recent skin irritation or trauma.

136 a) The chest X-ray shows a calcified pericardium. The echocardiogram shows a pericardial effusion inferiorly with fibrinous strands.

b) Tuberculosis, with constrictive pericarditis and pericardial effusion, respectively.

c) The second patient had HIV infection.

137 a) There is a penile ulcer with ipsilateral lymphadenopathy.

b) He had primary syphilis. Chancroid and lymphogranuloma venereum were excluded, and he remained HIV antibody negative on serial testing.

138 a) The patient has varicella (chickenpox).
   b) He is at risk from dissemination and visceral involvement, including varicella hepatitis, pneumonitis and encephalitis.
   c) He should be treated with intravenous high-dose acyclovir.

139 a) Acute pharyngeal diphtheria. A gray–white pseudomembrane is visible.
   b) Diphtheria antitoxin should be administered, after a test dose, without waiting for bacteriological confirmation. Penicillin or erythromycin are given to eradicate the organism.
   c) Culture of the organism and in-vitro testing for toxin production.

140 a) There is a complex tissue track extending from the right groin down to the psoas, which contains an abscess.
   b) A positive femoral stretch test and/or discharge of pus from the groin injection site.

141 a) He has schistosomiasis. The eggs in the upper figure have the terminal spines of *Schistosoma haematobium*. The ejaculate specimen (lower) contains numerous erythrocytes and white cells, and the ovum has hatched to yield a miracidium (the stage infective to the snail vector).

142 This man has had plombage (insertion of a biologically inert mass) to collapse part of his right lung, affected by tuberculosis in the pre-antibiotic era.

143 Kaposi's sarcoma affecting the oropharynx, including edema of the lips, and also involving the orbit and eye. AIDS.

144 a) Tick typhus.
   b) *Rickettsia conorii.*
   c) By the bite of an ixodid tick. The site of inoculation often forms a characteristic eschar, in this case in front of the ear.

145 There is a ragged stricture of the ileocecal region, with mucosal "thorn ulcers". The most likely radiological diagnosis is ileocecal tuberculosis, rather than Crohn's disease, amebiasis or yersiniosis.

146 a) The patient had Reiter's syndrome, with arthritis, conjunctivitis, circinate balanitis and urethritis.
   b) *Chlamydia trachomatis* was isolated on tissue culture of a urethral swab.

147 The patient has an unresolved atypical pneumonia. He should be asked about foreign travel (legionellosis), family respiratory illnesses (*Mycoplasma* infection) and contact with animals (Q fever) and birds (psittacosis). The patient was a bird fancier. A diagnosis of psittacosis was established serologically.

148 Possible pregnancy must be confirmed or excluded. If the pregnancy is confirmed, serological testing for recent rubella antibody must be undertaken immediately. It is helpful to establish whether the patient knows her rubella vaccination or antibody status. A past history of German measles is unreliable. Parvovirus B19 may cause a similar rash and is associated with fetal loss: antibody testing for this infection should be requested.

149 a) The film contains a single gametocyte of falciparum malaria. No ring forms were present. Apart from the characteristic shape and size of the parasite, its location within the erythrocyte distinguishes it from trypanosomes.

   b) Gametocytes may persist after treatment of malaria with schizonticidal drugs and are of no clinical significance to the patient. He only needs treatment with a gametocidal drug such as primaquine if he is living in a malaria-free region with mosquitoes capable of transmitting malaria, such as northern Australia.

150 a) There is gross retinal disruption and folding due to detachment.

   b) The prognosis is poor as conventional methods of retinal repair are hampered by background retinal damage due to CMV.

151 The tricuspid valve is the most common site of vegetations in association with endocarditis due to injecting drug abuse, as in this case. Infection acquired from intravenous central lines or pacemaker wires may also affect the tricuspid valve, and previous damage to the valve (e.g. rheumatic fever) will make infection more likely in any bacteremic patient.

152 There are extensive petechial lesions with early necrosis superimposed on edema. The picture suggests worsening of vasculitis rather than thrombocytopenia, and was probably precipitated by the interferon therapy.

153 a) There is a large calcified lesion in the spleen, typical of a long-standing hydatid cyst. Calcification of hematoma after trauma to the spleen is the main differential diagnosis.

   b) The cyst is likely to be parasitologically inert and is unlikely to grow any larger. In the absence of symptoms, no treatment (medical or surgical) is required.

154 a) It shows desquamation of the skin.

   b) In this context, the most likely diagnosis is toxic shock syndrome, caused by *Staphylococcus aureus* or *Streptococcus pyogenes*.

155 a) Primary herpes stomatitis with lesions on the tongue and lips.

   b) Electron microscopy and/or culture of swab from the lesion. In this case orogenitally acquired herpes simplex type II was confirmed.

   c) Oral acyclovir or famciclovir.

156 The myocardial tissue is partially replaced by inflammatory reaction. A cystic lesion containing dark staining organisms is also present, suggesting *Toxoplasma gondii* infection.

157 a) Apart from a small reactive right pleural effusion, there is bilateral apical calcification suggestive of previous tuberculosis, and there is a round opacity peripherally in the left mid zone. Ankylosing spondylitis is incidentally noted.

b) The peripheral lesion could be a tumor or tuberculoma. CT scan confirmed its peripheral location and guided needle biopsy showed it to be a tuberculoma.

158 This young man had opisthotonos due to tetanus. The most important differential diagnosis is meningitis. The commonest cause in developed countries is dystonic reactions due to anti-emetics such as meto-clopramide or prochlorperazine.

159 a) Streptococcal tonsillitis. The bilateral involvement suggests that infectious mononucleosis should be excluded.

b) Culture of throat swabs is less often successful than rapid agglu-tination tests for streptococcal antigens. Monospot or Paul-Bunnell tests would confirm glandular fever.

c) Penicillin (or erythromycin). Ampicillin derivatives should be avoided until EBV infection is excluded.

160 Extensive investigations failed to identify any focus of infection until a pelvic X-ray revealed chronic osteomyelitis of the right sacroiliac joint, the site of a previous injury.

161 a) Erysipelas, caused by infection with *Streptococcus pyogenes.*

b) Acute episodes respond readily to a penicillin or a macrolide antibiotic, but infection tends to recur from time to time, probably because of damaged lymphatics with impaired tissue drainage.

162 a) Calabar swelling.

b) Infection with the filaria, *Loa loa.*

c) Ivermectin is now the treatment of choice, superseding diethyl-carbamazine. Patients with very heavy infections may benefit from plasmapheresis to reduce filarial burden before chemotherapy.

163 a) Brucellosis (mainly *B. melitensis*) is common in the Middle East and serological tests and prolonged incubation of blood cultures (6 weeks) is indicated. Tuberculosis or other causes of chronic osteomyelitis should be considered.

b) He has scars of 'cupping' combined with scarification, and also has scars from cautery. These are commonly practiced by local healers.

164 a) The spleen is markedly enlarged and contains numerous small abscesses.

b) The most likely cause is *Mycobacterium avium* complex infection, and this was confirmed by blood and fecal cultures. The abscesses could have been aspirated.

165 a) It shows several worms in cross section, most probably *Strongyloides stercoralis* (confirmed by fecal microscopy).

   b) He should be treated with albendazole or ivermectin, which have superseded thiabendazole as the treatment of choice.

166 a) There is a rounded mass surrounded by a thin rim of air, within a larger apical mass. The likely diagnosis is an aspergilloma within an old tuberculous focus. Tumors may occasionally arise in the same location.

   b) Apart from general supportive care, surgical resection is often required.

167 a) Many sickle cells, nucleated red cells and toxic neutrophils.

   b) Pneumococcal septicemia is the most likely diagnosis and was confirmed in this case.

168 a) Cat scratch disease.

   b) *Bartonella* (formerly *Rochalimaea*) *hanselae* has been implicated as the usual cause, with a few cases ascribed to *Afipea felis*.

   c) None.

169 a) Chronic osteomyelitis.

   b) Secondary amyloidosis.

170 a) She had dengue fever. Scrub typhus and typhoid should be excluded as well as malaria (which does not produce this sort of rash).

   b) She settled on symptomatic therapy. Resolution is usually complete but some patients develop a prolonged fatigue state after infection.

171 a) Oral candidiasis.

   b) Such pronounced candidiasis is likely to be associated with immunosuppression and a short course of systemically absorbed treatment such as fluconazole or itraconazole would be appropriate. Topical nystatin, amphotericin B or clotrimazole could be used if these were not available. In patients with HIV, the risks and benefits of different secondary prophylaxis regimens are currently being debated.

172 a) A maggot of the tumbu fly, *Cordylobia anthropophaga,* is emerging from the lesion, in response to hypoxia induced by occlusion of the wound entrance by the petroleum jelly (the treatment of choice).

   b) Clothes that have been washed should be ironed carefully to kill eggs deposited by flies.

173 a) Meningococcal meningitis.

   b) In Africans the rash of meningococcal disease may have a papular component and may be palpable even if difficult to visualize on a very dark skin. The conjunctivae should also be carefully examined.

174 a) Several thin-walled abscesses are visible without fluid levels.

b) In the context of the history given, a Gram negative infection from the urinary tract is most likely. *Pseudomonas aeruginosa* was cultured from urine, blood and sputum. The patient responded well to prolonged ceftazidime therapy.

175 a) There are a few giant cells and yeast-like organisms are visible. Mucicarmine selectively stains the capsule of *Cryptococcus* sp., distinguishing it from *Candida* sp. and *Histoplasma* sp.

b) Parenteral amphotericin B, followed by maintenance therapy with an imidazole such as fluconazole.

176 a) There is widening of the aortic arch which contains curvilinear calcification, suggestive of a syphilitic aortic aneurysm.

b) Reaginic and specific tests for syphilis were positive.

c) Penicillin treatment may induce acute inflammation and obstruction of the coronary ostia, with myocardial insufficiency. The risk is reduced if the patient is given steroids before antibiotic therapy starts.

177 a) Vasculitic/purpuric lesions on the sole of one foot.

b) *Staphylococcus aureus* is the usual pathogen when lesions are as florid as this.

c) The unilateral location suggests a focal infection in the blood supply to one leg, for example infected vascular graft. In this instance, infection arose from an infected femoral pseudoaneurysm due to injecting drug abuse. Endocarditis should still be excluded.

178 a) There are numerous open abscesses extending above and below both inguinal ligaments. There is also a macular rash on the abdomen.

b) Chancroid was initially considered as well as tuberculosis. *Mycobacterium tuberculosis* was cultured. The abdominal rash followed treatment with cotrimoxazole. The patient was HIV positive.

Index